Minerals: Kill or Cure?

by Ruth Adams
and
Frank Murray

Larchmont Books
NEW YORK

MINERALS: KILL OR CURE?

Second printing: January 1977.
First printing: July 1974.

ISBN 0-915962-16-0

Printed in United States of America

LARCHMONT BOOKS
6 East 43rd Street
New York, N.Y. 10017

Contents

Foreword

THE "WELL-BALANCED MEAL," so often prescribed and so rarely obtained, has fats, carbohydrates, proteins, vitamins and minerals. The basic building blocks for our tissues, and the source of energy for our organs, are the fats, carbohydrates and proteins. The vitamins and minerals are essential in the chemical processes which convert these three types of foods into our tissues, and our energy.

Over a hundred years ago, physicians were describing the need for good nutrition for physical and mental health. As the years progressed, "good nutrition" became more defined. Food was divided into the three classes and the need for all three types of food was recognized. Later, vitamins were discovered and the science of nutrition expanded in an exciting manner. As vitamins were isolated, and experiments on the development of diseases caused by lack of vitamins were done, new words were added to the vocabulary: beriberi, scurvy and pellagra—all vitamin-deficiency diseases. More recently, vitamins have been used in massive doses to treat such diseases as schizophrenia. The understanding and the use of vitamins continues to expand.

Perhaps the relative ease in working with vitamins, the lack of tremendously complicated interaction between vitamins—the excitement of a new discovery—explains why vitamins were in the spotlight in the nutritional field for so long. In any event, minerals are beginning to usurp that spotlight. Although minerals have been listed on the table of elements for all to see, they have not been given their proper importance until recently. The last 10 years has seen an upsurge in the basic science research on minerals. Ruth Adams and Frank Murray have presented, in "Minerals: Kill or Cure?" an excellent survey of minerals, their importance in nutrition, the dangers of mineral pollution, the complicated interrelation of minerals, and many valuable references. All of this information and their straight-forward presentation make this book uniquely adapted to the professional and non-professional reader. From knowledge gained through this text, the reader will have sufficient background to follow the important discoveries that the following years will add to our understanding of the minerals in human nutrition, in health and disease.

HARVEY M. ROSS, M.D.
May, 1974
West Hollywood, California

CHAPTER 1

Minerals and Trace Minerals—Mysterious and Essential

ACCORDING TO THE National Institutes of Health, Bethesda, Maryland, the mature human body is the end result of nearly 20 years of growth. Each individual begins as the product of two cells and eventually is made up of 100,000 billion cells. The most rapid and crucial period of growth in the human being occurs in the nine months before birth.

Every minute in the human body, three billion cells die and three billion cells are created. Every one of these cells contains protein, which must be obtained from the food you eat. Carbohydrates and fats cannot provide the building material for cells. It must be protein and the only source of such protein is high-protein food. Involved with the protein in this rebuilding process are vitamins, minerals and enzymes, as well as an unknown number of other substances, all of which are present in natural food and drinking water. When human cells become malnourished or malformed—because of an improper diet, air and water pollution, too many chemicals in our food supply, etc.—this becomes a precursor for a long list of degenerative disorders.

For the purpose of this book, we are confining our discussion primarily to minerals. We will be reviewing some of the latest research involving the six essential minerals for which there are recommended dietary allowances (calcium, phosphorus, iodine, iron, zinc and magnesium); and trace minerals necessary for human health (copper, chromium, manganese, molybdenum, selenium, sodium, potassium, etc.); and trace metals which have some bearing on human nutrition (lithium, silver, nickel, barium, boron, etc.) We will also explain why some trace minerals are harmful to humans, especially when taken in excessive amounts (fluorine, cadmium, lead, mercury, sodium, etc.).

The Food and Drug Administration tells us repeatedly that "the average American diet" is the best in the world and that, nutritionally speaking, we've never been so well nourished. In fact, the FDA was once so bold as to suggest that the following legend appear on all food supplement labels: "Vitamins and minerals are supplied in abundant amounts by the food we eat . . . Dietary needs should be satisfied by foods. Except for persons with special medical needs, there is no scientific basis for recommending use of dietary supplements."

Obviously, this statement is untrue. As we will explore, the U. S. Department of Agriculture, the U. S. Public Health Service, testimony before the U. S. Senate Select Committee on Nutrition and Human Needs, and independent nutrition surveys demonstrate that many Americans, regardless of income, are malnourished. In the meantime, scientists around the world are delving deeper into the mysterious way in which minerals affect human nutrition. And much of this research, as we will see, is as exciting as that currently being done with vitamins.

All living things contain a variety of minerals. Some occur in such small amounts that early chemical analyses could barely detect them. They, therefore, became known as the trace minerals, metals or elements. Although only a relatively few of these more than 100 elements have nutritional requirements or biological functions, it is likely that many of the others occur in living things only by accident, having been acquired in the food or water, or absorbed through the skin, or even inhaled.

"At the present stage of our biological knowledge, we cannot ignore the possibility that some of the trace elements we now think of as nonessential do have as yet unrecognized functions in the body's processes," *Food*, the Yearbook of Agriculture, tells us.

"People found out about the need for trace elements when they saw that some deficiency diseases in livestock, and sometimes in human beings, could be treated by large doses of a specific mineral.

"An example is iodine, which was used in a somewhat hit-or-miss way to treat goiter as long ago as 1820. A study of the distribution of iodine in soils and water later led to the belief that goiter often is a nutritional disease, especially in places where the natural supply of iodine is low. Scientists in 1895 proved that iodine is a normal component of the thyroid gland and is depleted in cases of endemic goiter. Today we recognize iodine as a component of the hormones produced by the thyroid gland."

Food goes on to state that cobalt is another example. "Investigators in 1935 discovered that this element prevented certain wasting diseases of sheep and cattle in localities in Australia and New Zealand. Subsequent studies demonstrated that a deficiency of cobalt was responsible for similar diseases in Florida, parts of England and Scotland, and Kenya. As with iodine, the function of cobalt remained obscure for some time after the need for it in animal nutrition was recognized."

Scientists have known for some time that some trace minerals are essential for health and others are harmful. However, says a review in *Science* for July 20, 1973, "Only very recently have most scientists begun to appreciate the full extent and the great complexity of the interactions between environmental trace elements and human health."

The *Science* article by Thomas H. Maugh II summarizes the papers presented at a recent conference on the effect of trace minerals on health. "The time may be fast approaching," says Dr. Maugh, "when evaluation of trace elements concentrations will play a fundamental role in the diagnosis of illness and when manipulation of those concentrations may play an even greater role in prevention."

At last count, 14 trace minerals were judged to be essential to human health. One of these is fluoride, which some scientists declare is essential to life, while others point out that it may be harmful in some ways to human health, although it apparently does prevent (or perhaps delay a bit) the onset of tooth decay.

Dr. H. A. Schroeder of Dartmouth Medical School, one of the giants in the field of trace mineral research, has accumulated considerable evidence showing that heart disease tends to be less prevalent in communities where the drinking water contains many minerals. This suggests, incidentally, that using softened water for drinking is not wise, since most of these naturally occurring minerals are removed in the softening process and sodium replaces them.

Researchers have found that as many as 43 trace elements may be ingredients of tooth enamel. Recently it has been suggested that some of these may help to prevent decay: molybdenum, vanadium, boron, strontium, barium, lithium, titanium and aluminum. Getting too much lead, copper, zinc and chromium may tend to increase the tooth's susceptibility to decay.

We know that the trace mineral cadmium is an increasingly plentiful pollutant in many parts of the world where air pollution from fuels burned and manufacturing plants releases cadmium into the air. This mineral is suspected of being part of the reason for high blood pressure in these areas. In addition, it is known that cadmium pollution causes fragile bones. In an area of Japan, a disease which affected many people in the 1950's was called the "ouch-ouch" disease because of the very painful bone condition it induced. A nearby factory had been discharging cadmium into the river from which drinking water was drawn. Quite recently, the residents of this locality were compensated financially for the damage done to their health by cadmium pollution.

Other seemingly strange things happened involving trace metals. Sheep which grazed beneath high voltage power lines became poisoned by getting too much copper. Tests of the ground beneath the wires showed more than twice the copper of nearby fields. But why did other copper cables not produce the same kind of pollution? It is suspected that the air pollution in this industrial area was releasing sulfur dioxide which, in turn, eroded the copper from the wires.

Most fascinating is a study by Dr. Maurice L. Sievers of the Phoenix Indian Medical Center, Arizona, who has studied the trace minerals to which Indians of that area are exposed. Drinking water contains sodium, chlorine, calcium, magnesium, strontium, boron, lithium and molybdenum. It is deficient in the usual amounts of copper, zinc and manganese. Foods raised on the reservation also tend to concentrate various trace minerals. Mesquite beans concentrate strontium; cabbages accumulate sulfate; a certain local berry contains almost unbelievable amounts of lithium. Indians on the reservation have a less than average incidence of hardening of the arteries and high blood preasure. Is this because of the calcium and magnesium in the water? Or can the lack of hardening of the arteries and heart attacks be caused by the lithium in the drinking water? These are provocative questions which further study of trace minerals is bound to solve eventually.

Other intriguing aspects of the trace metals story

involve selenium which, under some circumstances, is beneficial and at other times harmful. Giving selenium to animals on a low protein diet resulted in damage to their hearts and livers and threw off the balance of other trace minerals: magnesium, copper and manganese. Adding cobalt to this test made all the changes worse.

Some time ago medical scientists were very alarmed over something called "beer drinkers' cardiomyopathy", which produced deaths in people drinking beer, presumably because of the cobalt used to stabilize the foam. Now a Nebraska researcher feels certain that the cobalt was not alone responsible, but that the cobalt became toxic only because of the selenium already in the beer. These are intriguing mysteries which much further research is needed to clarify.

A Soviet Union scientist sent a paper to the same conference reporting that certain kinds of medicinal herbs concentrate helpful trace minerals and so are being used to treat some kinds of heart disease. At similar conferences in the past, evidence has been presented showing that "the weeds"—the wayside herbs, that is, with their deep roots—may be sources of many trace minerals which they bring up from far below the surface where the roots of most garden plants do not go.

So there seem to be two main reasons for studying trace elements and using all our knowledge of them for better health: first, we need to know which are toxic to human beings and how to avoid them in industrial pollution. Then we need to know much, much more about the helpful ones—which ones we need, how much we need and in what combinations with other minerals and trace minerals. There seems to be no doubt that we can eventually discover much that will be helpful to human health.

Meanwhile, what can we non-scientists do to assure ourselves that we are getting all the trace minerals we should have in proper proportions so far as present

CHAPTER 2

The Importance of Trace Elements in Your Diet

UNTIL QUITE RECENTLY scientists paid little attention to the subject of trace minerals. Nobody knew exactly which of them, if any, were essential for life and which were just contaminants we'd be better off without. Nor was there any exact way to study them, since some of them seem to be ever-present in air and water, so that experiments designed to see what happens when they are absent just couldn't be worked out. And besides, the American food supply is presumed to be so well planned that all our requirements for trace elements should be easily met.

Now, we are glad to say, interest in trace metals is very high. An article in the *Journal of the American Medical Association* asked, "How Important Are Trace Elements in Diet?" The article discussed three important findings in regard to three trace minerals: copper, zinc and chromium. We don't hear much about these in newspaper and magazine articles on nutrition because it is generally taken for granted that all of us get enough of them in our food. Let's see.

At a Puerto Rican Nutrition Congress, a Peruvian doctor claimed that a copper deficiency is a "real, existing, pathological entity." Dr. Angel Cordano said that it should be looked for in severely malnourished children, in those which have a chronic inability to absorb food properly and in premature infants.

In his study of 178 malnourished children, he found that 60 of them developed some signs of copper deficiency during a hospital stay while they were kept on a diet poor in copper. Twenty of them had symptoms of deficiency when they came to the hospital. In the case of premature infants or those whose birth weight is very low, an exclusive milk diet for more than four months is likely to produce a deficiency in copper.

In a laboratory experiment with rats, it was found that deficiency in zinc will result in gross malformations among most of the young, when mothers are kept on diets deficient in zinc throughout pregnancy. Litters were smaller and the birth weight was lower, as well. Malformations included such things as cleft palate, club foot, heart and lung deformities and many more. The mother rats apparently could not use zinc from their own bodies' supplies to give to their developing infants. We do not know as yet whether the same is true of human mothers.

A Food and Drug Administration researcher, Dr. Leon L. Hopkins, used chromium in experiments with middle-aged human volunteers whose blood sugar levels were not normal, although they were not diabetic. An estimated 40 per cent of middle-aged Americans are believed to have such an impairment of their blood sugar regulating mechanism, although they are also not diabetic.

Small doses of chromium were given to the volunteers every day for two months and almost all of them had a downward trend in the blood sugar reading. Those who did not respond were the overweight ones. Volunteers with normal blood sugar levels took the chromium with no noticeable effects.

> **Zinc deficiency (in soils) is more common world-wide than that of any other trace element. . . . In the USA zinc deficiency is known in 32 different states. . . . Over forty different crops have been found zinc deficient. —"A Mine to Market Outline—Zinc," published by the American Zinc Institute.**

Says the *Journal of the American Medical Association*, reporting this astonishing experiment performed by an FDA scientist: "Dr. Hopkins' study supports the work of other investigators who have reported normalization of glucose tolerance tests in response to chromium supplementation. Such a response has been observed in 40 per cent of elderly Americans with moderate impairment and 50 percent of selected patients who have maturity onset diabetes with severely impaired glucose tolerances." They quote Dr. Hopkins as saying that daily supplements of chromium could improve the blood sugar condition of almost 13 million people in the United States. These include people with no evidence of diabetes and about 25 to 50 per cent of certain cases of diabetes, as well.

Dr. Hopkins goes on to point out that adding chromium to foods would be the answer. "People may soon want to start putting chromium into such food as flour and salt," he says. So the FDA is proceeding with experiments to test the complete safety of chromium used in this way as a food supplement.

"Over the last 100 years, and especially in the last 30 years, a steadily increasing number of elements has been found to be constantly present in living tissues. To a few of them, definite biological functions have been assigned. The term 'trace elements' was quite understandably applied by the early workers to those elements which occur, or which function, in very small amounts relative to the amounts of the main constituents of the tissues, because of the difficulties then associated with measuring the low concentrations involved and their recognition, therefore, merely as 'traces.'"

The words are those of E. J. Underwood of the Institute of Agriculture, University of West Australia, in his book *Trace Elements*. He reminds us that, although the term "trace" implies extremely small amounts, this does not mean that those minerals are lacking in importance.

Nearly every chemical element has been found to occur in living tissues at some time or another, he says. One of the earliest investigators found in human blood: silver, aluminium, copper, iron, magnesium, manganese, calcium, phosphorus, silicon, titanium and zinc. Later rubidium and lithium were added to this list. Iodine, cobalt, molybdenum, nickel, chromium, tin, lead, arsenic, fluorine, bromine, selenium, boron, barium and strontium have also been found in tissues of plants and animals.

Some of these (iron, copper, manganese, zinc, iodine and cobalt) are definitely established as essential for the health of living things. Plants apparently do not require iodine and cobalt to be healthy. They *do* require boron and silicon, which perhaps animals, including man, do not need. Just knowing that one or another of the trace minerals is present in our cells does not mean necessarily that we require it to live. It may be there simply because it exists in our food and so our bodies have developed what Dr. Underwood calls a "passive tolerance" to it. But he feels sure that, as time goes on, more and more of these will be found to be essential to us, rather than just something that happens to be present.

Aside from the fact that they are grouped together and called "trace elements," these minerals have little in common. We need some of them in far greater amounts than we need others. For instance, a certain amount of whole blood may contain only 8-12 micrograms of iodine but 50,000 micrograms of iron. We need that much more of iron.

One of the ways in which investigators became aware of the importance of the trace minerals was when they began to investigate naturally occurring diseases of man, which were widely separated geographically, and showed that they might be due to a deficiency or an excess of one or another of the trace minerals. The classic example is that lack of iodine in food and water in certain regions of the world is the primary cause of goiter in both man and animals. On the other hand, too much of molybdenum in the soil can result in a disease of cattle.

Says Dr. Underwood, "Soil-plant-animal interrelationships were given added meaning and significance, especially as the soil deficiencies or excesses primarily responsible for the disease condition in animals sometimes affected plant growth or health as well as plant composition." In other words, researchers became aware of the fact that the trace mineral exists first in the soil, then in the plant, then in the animal or human that eats the plant. Too little or too much of some mineral may adversely affect the health of the plant. The plant may be

---

Chromium Content of Some Sugars and Fats

Here is a comparison of the amount of the trace mineral chromium in some sugars and some fats:

	Micrograms of chromium
Sugar, white refined	none
Raw sugar	1.59
Brown sugar	1.19
Maple syrup	3.07
Corn oil	1.64 to 2.31
Cottonseed oil	1.64 to 2.31
Sunflower seed oil	1.11
Soy lecithin	4.17

H. A. Schroeder, in *Circulation*, March, 1967

Zinc and Chromium Content of Some Common Foods

Here is a comparison of the zinc and chromium content of wheat, white flour, bran and wheat germ.

	Zinc mcg	Chromium mcg
Wheat	31.5	0.97
Patent flour	8.9	0.58
Bran	100.2	1.24
Germ	133.4	1.36

H. A. Schroeder, in *Circulation*, March, 1967

---

able to flourish without some other mineral, whereas the animal or person who eats it may get into trouble because the balance of trace minerals it contains is not right for *him*.

But the relationship is not nearly so simple as it sounds, says Dr. Underwood. There may be more subtle, milder forms of deficiency, less dramatic, and these may be determined by the extent to which other food elements are lacking in the diet. Vitamins, for instance, combine with the trace minerals to make "enzyme systems" for processing fats, proteins and carbohydrates. Lack of a vitamin might have something to do with the amount of a certain trace mineral you need or do not need.

In general, the trace minerals seem to function as "catalysts"—that is, substances which cause certain things to take place, without themselves being permanently affected or used up in the process. As an example, iodine is an extremely important part of thyroxin, a hormone manufactured by the thyroid gland. This hormone brings about powerful reactions in many different parts of the body. And there can be no hormone if iodine is not present in the food eaten.

You can readily see what the consequences are when whole communities eat food grown on soil deficient in iodine. The plants are perfectly healthy, crops do not suffer. But the people and animals who eat the plants develop, first, goiters, which are enlargements of the thyroid gland and, in serious deficiencies, children are born stunted physically and mentally. Nervous systems, eyes and reproductive systems are affected.

The largest amounts of zinc present in human bodies, as we will discuss in more detail in a later chapter, are concentrated in bones, teeth, pancreas and male reproductive organs. Zinc is also present in the colored parts of the eye. Some researchers believe that this metal may be related to the color of hair. One cannot help but speculate about the possible relation of zinc deficiency in diet to the many disorders that harass present-day Americans.

In *New Scientist* for April 5, 1962, an Australian scientist discusses the lack of trace minerals in soils in wide areas of Australia. Copper, zinc and molybdenum are the minerals which are critically deficient. Supplying these has made fertile millions of acres of land that formerly could not be cultivated. Lack of cobalt and copper is the cause of a mysterious disease which afflicted sheep and cattle in certain areas of Australia, as we have mentioned. Giving cobalt in extremely small amounts means the difference between life and death. K. Loftus Hill, author of the *New Scientist* article, tells us that only one ounce of cobalt will keep 800 sheep healthy for 12 months.

Apart from its association with cobalt, copper deficiency causes certain very serious conditions in Australian livestock when it alone is lacking. One of these is sudden death from heart failure. The cattle suffer first from anemia, which exists only during the spring months. It disappears suddenly during the summer, even though the concentration of copper in the blood remains very low. Then, over a period of several years, the heart condition apparently becomes worse and, finally, the animal dies suddenly with a heart attack. No one knows why a deficiency in copper should cause such a condition. Could not the same deficiency cause sudden human heart attacks?

Harry V. Warren, Professor of Minerology at the University of British Columbia, writing in the *Canadian Journal of Public Health*, April 1961, tells us he has been studying the amounts of trace minerals in soil, trying to find a "normal" composition which could be recommended as the best possible mixture of these important elements for the good of the plant and also the animal eating the plant. He says, "We have encountered numerous variations from the normal, variations so great that we came to the conclusion that if such anomalies (deviations) extended to vegetables being eaten by animals or men it must affect their health."

The source of minerals in soils is the rock foundation under the soil. Dr. Warren has found that multiple sclerosis is very common in certain parts of the world, which are quite close to other localities where the disease is not common. What could make the difference? The trace minerals in the soil could. In areas where there is little multiple sclerosis, there is a rock formation which would provide very little lead in the soil. In other areas where there is considerable lead in the soil, MS is more prevalent. Are those facts related? No one knows, but the opportunities for further investigation are fascinating. Does our present incidence of multiple sclerosis have anything to do with the high lead contamination of the air in our cities?

Listen to what Dr. Warren has to say about the relation of trace elements to health: "Medical men have long known that trace elements and particularly metals such as copper, lead, molybdenum, silver, mercury and cadmium play an important role in determining the health of animals and humans. Agriculturists have realized that trace elements vitally affect the health both of agricultural crops and of the animals and humans that eat these crops. Although there is a wealth of information on the trace element content of foods, the information usually deals only with foods grown over normal soils. There are just enough anomalous areas in various parts of the world to justify attempts to discover what does happen when these . . . areas produce food crops and these crops find their way into our food supplies."

These days, almost anyone who believes that our present-day food may be deficient in important trace minerals is called a "food faddist" and ridiculed. As we will see throughout this book, there are many experts who will agree with us that we are not always getting the proper amounts of vitamins and minerals from our food.

One can conclude only that many of us may be suffering from deficiencies in trace minerals because of any or all of the following reasons:

1. Peculiar food habits. There are plenty of people who just never eat enough unrefined cereals, vegetables and fruits, which are the richest sources of most of the trace minerals.

2. Refining and processing, as we will mention often in this book, may deplete our cereal foods of almost all their trace elements. For instance, white bread contains no noticeable amounts of zinc or magnesium. Manganese exists almost entirely in the bran of the cereal. Whole wheat flour contains more than six times as much as white flour.

3. Certainly the very small amount of evidence we have given above shows the relation between depleted soil and the mineral content of food. We are using our farmland to produce crops of unprecedented abundance. We are replenishing in the soil only those minerals which occur in large amounts—calcium, phosphorus and potas-

sium. The loss of trace minerals from cropping and from soil erosion is ignored. The organic farmer and gardener, on the other hand, restore trace minerals by giving their soil large amounts of organic fertilizer.

The most effective argument for organic gardening and farming, it seems to us, is that the natural, organic fertilizers used in this ancient way of growing things restore to the soil trace minerals which are likely to become exhausted if only the usual commercial fertilizers are used.

As we stated, the commercial, chemically formulated fertilizers consist of measured amounts of mostly three minerals. Sometimes other minerals are mixed in for special needs. Agricultural experts who do not favor organic gardening, and those who work for the big agri-chemical business, tell us constantly that these are the only minerals the plants need. Using these minerals and nothing else will produce ample crops, they say, and the plants will have all the nutriment they need.

Granted that this may be so in most cases, we would argue that we are not as interested in the health of garden plants as in the health of human beings. And if it is possible to raise plants using only a limited few minerals, it's quite possible that these healthy plants will not contain enough of all the trace minerals to make healthy people out of those of us who eat the produce.

Common sense tells you that taking one crop after another off a given acreage of land year after year reduces the trace minerals in that soil. How could it not, if you do not replenish these minerals by fertilization? So the organic farmer, using ground corn cobs, compost, leaves, grass clippings, hay, straw mulches, cover crops chopped and plowed into his soil, restores to the soil the abundance of trace minerals that exist in these many, varied kinds of natural fertilizers.

Officially we are told that there is no such thing as soil deficiency in the United States. In the August 1968 issue of *Today's Health,* which is published by the American Medical Association, this letter appeared: "Is the nutrient value of food affected by the soil on which it grows?" Their answer: "Within certain limits, the nutrient content of crops can be affected by the soil on which they are grown. . . . In this country, however, there is no documented evidence to indicate that these variations significantly affect human nutrition. . . ."

So the nutrients in any given mouthful of food can be affected by the presence or absence of minerals in the soil in which it was grown. For a long time there was no "documented evidence" as to the importance of iodine in the soil to prevent goiter. Now it is an accepted nutritional fact.

Sailors hailing from three areas of the United States were found to be completely free from tooth cavities, according to *The New York Times,* December 18, 1967. The locations were northwestern Ohio, west central Florida and northeastern South Carolina. The Office of Naval Research stated that such a finding must mean "there is something in the water and soil of these three areas which combines with fluoride to provide increased protection against tooth decay."

What could it be, if not minerals? And how will the FDA and the Public Health Service continue to justify their point of view, if, indeed, it is shown that freedom from tooth decay results from minerals in the soil which the rest of us don't get in our food?

And the *Journal of Dental Research* has printed an article by two researchers showing that cereals from different geographic areas produce different amounts of tooth decay. In the experiments performed in a laboratory, the scientists exposed tooth enamel to different grains: wheat, corn, oats and barley, all grown in different states. Flour from California dissolved more enamel than that from other states. Iowa flour produced much less decay than that from Texas and Canada. But whole

CHAPTER 3

Trace Minerals—
Friend or Foe?

"THE POSSIBILITY OF causal relationships between environmental factors and the occurrence of many degenerative diseases is slowly being recognized," reports Helen L. Cannon of the U.S. Geological Survey in Denver, Colorado, and Howard C. Hopps of the University of Missouri. They were writing in the December 11, 1970 issue of *Science*.

"One aspect of the environment—that concerned with geochemistry of rocks, soil, plants and water—should be studied carefully and the distribution of minor elements be compared with geographic patterns of animal and human health and disease," the scientists continue. "We know that calcium, phosphorus, iron, copper and all the other important inorganic nutrients somehow make their way from a never-ending source in the rocks that form our continents to the soils and waters, and from there into plants, animals and, finally man.

"But many questions come to mind. How is this transport accomplished and how easily do the various elements move into and through the food chain? What effects do climate and time have on this movement? What sort of interactions go on between the various elements as they come into contact with one another to enhance or hinder this process? How are these elements utilized by different kinds of organisms and what effects do even small excesses or deficiencies of any one ion have on the health of plants or animals?"

One of the most important aspects of the extent of our ignorance of trace minerals is demonstrated in an article by W. G. Hoekstra of the University of Wisconsin in *Federation Proceedings* for September-October, 1964. After reviewing many angles of the various relationships between phosphorus and calcium, between zinc and calcium, and between zinc and copper, cadmium, iron, molybdenum, Dr. Hoekstra says, "The complexity of the mineral imbalance problem is apparent." He concludes by saying, "It is apparent that our understanding of the mechanisms of mineral imbalances is fragmentary. New interrelationships are constantly being discovered. It is my firm opinion that we are presently recognizing and correcting only a small fraction of the mineral imbalance problems currently plaguing animals and man."

In the Winter 1972 issue of the *Journal of Applied Nutrition,* John J. Miller, Ph.D., speaks of the relation of minerals to preventive medicine. He mentions the pioneering work of Drs. Evan and Wilfrid Shute in Canada on vitamin E and Dr. Linus Pauling's book on *Vitamin C and the Common Cold,* then goes on to say, "understanding the importance of these great vitamin discoveries by such progressive scientists is not enough. We, therefore, add a strong plea for an appreciation of the role of essential minerals in the metabolic reactions of all human and animal bodies. And by this statement I do not mean merely that we should admit their value in a superficial way. Rather we must eagerly learn to the greatest extent just how they function and why they are so essential in every part of the organism."

He tells us that minerals and trace minerals are engaged in the movements of every muscle, in the genetic transmission of traits from one generation to another and "the harmony or lack of harmony of thoughts flashing through the brain." He asks why physicians almost entirely ignore this important aspect of good health. Laboratories do not usually test for anything other than calcium, phosphorus, sodium and potassium in cases of brain or nerve disorders, for example. Tests even for these show nothing much more than what minerals are circulating in the blood or what has been lost in the urine. Tests for magnesium, zinc, iron and manganese are too expensive. And, apart from iron, no one knows exactly what they do in the body—so how could they tell whether or not they are performing their proper function?

Dr. Miller gives an example of a 60-year-old man who came to a hospital complaining of being chronically miserable and mentally discouraged. He had been hospitalized and tested for two years—at a cost of $10,000. He had been told he had low blood sugar and a "questionable" heart condition. The patient dutifully followed the prescribed diet and continued to become worse. Further tests were then done on other minerals. It was discovered that he was excreting magnesium and potassium in amounts that were much too high. And, finally, when a sample of hair was tested, it was found to contain 2,380 parts per million of lead. Dr. Miller tells us that this great overburden of lead could have disrupted the body activity of all these trace minerals: calcium, magnesium, iron, potassium, sodium and zinc.

The tests also showed that levels of potassium were very low in relation to zinc—and this indicates low blood sugar, which is aggravated, according to Dr. Miller, by a low ratio of manganese to lead and a high ratio of calcium to potassium. All these intricacies demonstrate what you get into when you upset natural mineral balances. Since we do not have even the vaguest idea of what these interrelationships may be, in most cases, every new environmental pollutant carries the potential for upsetting a whole maze of interrelationships among trace minerals in the body. And every new crop taken off soil which is fertilized only with fertilizer containing three or four basic minerals—and no more—can, conceivably, bring about still greater imbalances in body minerals. What the results will be in the form of poor health are anyone's guess.

"The neglect of nutrition by the public in general is largely responsible for the huge increase in cost of health care in the United States—jumping from $12 billion in 1950 to $75 billion in 1971," reports Dr. Miller. "And if present estimates should prove to be correct, the figure will be $105 billion in 1974—which means a 900 per cent increase. Surely some way must be found to avoid the increases in the public debt thus involved, for the burden of the taxes that most citizens are now faced to pay is stress that seriously affects their physical and mental well being. Such economic conditions, together with a rapidly deteriorating environment throughout the entire land, have become a threat to the health of our people."

How does "the average American" fare in regard to trace minerals when he is placed on any kind of special diet, for whatever reason? The answer is given in an article in *Journal of the American Dietetic Association*, May 1970. Dr. Annette Gormican of the Department of Medicine and Nutritional Sciences, University of Wisconsin, dealt with menus planned for patients in hospitals. Dieticians and doctors involved in these "special diet" programs rely on official tables of the nutrient content of foods, taking for granted that, while there may be some discrepancies, the foods will, in general, average out to about the same amounts as these tables show.

Dr. Gormican analyzed 128 foods served in hospital meals. She studied the following minerals: calcium, phosphorus, potassium, magnesium, sodium, aluminum, barium, iron, strontium, boron, copper, zinc, manganese and chromium. She found that there is a wide range of discrepancies in the trace mineral content of common foods, compared to the official tables. Iron and copper varied widely. In some cases, they were higher than the official levels; in some cases lower.

The fresh, home-grown tomatoes used in this hospital were lower in calcium, phosphorus, potassium, sodium and iron than the amounts recorded as official in the U. S. Agriculture Handbook, *Composition of Foods*. A large amount of aluminum was found in one kind of processed cheese. The reason? It contains an emulsifier, permitted by law, which is sodium aluminum phosphate.

"It is generally accepted," says Dr. Gormican, "that trace elements in food vary considerably because of locality and contamination." She means, we presume, the chemical additives, which are added either intentionally, as with the emulsifier, or unintentionally, as with pesticides, fertilizers and the thousands of other chemicals which get into food one way or another.

Comparing the hospital diets with those studied by other workers in this field, Dr. Gormican found that "Much lower values were observed for magnesium, aluminum, barium, iron, boron, copper and manganese. The levels of phosphorus, potassium, calcium, sodium and zinc were just about the same as those listed in 'the average American diet' by other scientists. In the case of chromium, the level appeared to be a bit higher."

Dr. Gormican tells us that some of the diets in the hospital were 1,000-calorie diets, 1,500-calorie diets, "soft" diets, low-sodium diets, diets containing only 40 grams of protein instead of the 50 or so grams recommended for healthy adults, diets containing only 20 grams of protein, full liquid diets, clear liquid diets, and so on. These were some of the diets being eaten by patients in this hospital.

Compare this with the "Total diet" study which involves a mythical, healthy 18-year-old boy eating 4,200 calories a day—more than four times as much as some of these patients were eating. A diet containing only 20 grams of protein could not maintain a healthy person. How could it possibly provide what is needed for a sick person when illness, a form of stress, vastly increases all of one's nutritional needs? The "Total diet," incidentally, was the brain child of the U. S. Department of Agriculture. Carefully selecting the foods they *thought* an 18-year-old boy would eat from the local supermarket (rather than the hot dogs, potato chips, donuts and soft drinks that most 18-year-olds consume), USDA experts set up diet guidelines which were supposed to be valid for all of us, regardless of age, physical condition, etc.

What were some of the foods eaten by the patients studied by Dr. Gormican? For someone who has lived with good, sound nutrition practices for many years, some of the foods listed by these patients boggle the mind. They contain almost nothing of nutritional value—and here they are being presented on hospital trays, by trained dieticians, to people whose every bite of food must be measured in terms of nutritional content.

Are you ready? Cheerios, corn flakes, saltines, noodles, macaroni, puffed rice, rice crispies, white rice, spaghetti, sugar (brown, white and powdered), and white, bleached flour. In addition, the patients were served meat, milk, eggs, cheese, fruits and vegetables. These latter foods are, of course, nourishing and whole. They are the only foods that should be served to anyone, well or ill, along with real, whole-grain cereals and breads. Diluting an already seriously limited diet (such as 1,000 calories, 20 grams of protein) with foods that contain almost nothing but empty calories is simply unforgivable when a well person is involved. How much more catastrophic it becomes when the people being fed are ill!

The hospital diet is a very typical American diet, high in refined cereals and sugar, and lacking entirely in those vegetable foods which contain the most minerals and trace minerals, as well as vitamins and protein: the whole grains and whole cereals, nuts, seeds, wheat germ, wheat bran. Is it any wonder our hospital beds are full? Is it any wonder patients emerging from such an institution require long convalescent periods? Is it any wonder many trace minerals were found to be deficient in such a diet?

But what about those of us who are not in hospitals? Are we getting enough—or too much—of the minerals and trace minerals? In *Mining Engineering* for July 1962, Dr. Harry V. Warren, Professor of Geology at the University of British Columbia, quoted these words of Dr. Henry Schroeder: "It is a fascinating hypothesis that some of the chronic and fatal ailments of human beings may be the result of accumulations, deficiencies or displacements of certain trace metals." It seems that this is still a hypothesis, but, in the 11 years since then, we have come a short way toward comprehending some of these complexities.

For example, trace elements in soil and water appear to have something to do with incidence of heart and artery problems. Hansford Shacklette of the U. S. Geological Survey in Denver, Colorado, as reported in the *American Geology Society Bulletin* (83(4) 1077-1082, 1972), did a study of nine counties in Georgia which have varying amounts of trace minerals. The greater amounts of trace minerals in soil occur in those counties which have the lowest figures for heart attacks.

Trace minerals enter into both local food and water supplies. So it appears that more, rather than less, of trace minerals in general promise greater freedom from heart problems. This would certainly suggest not using distilled drinking water, since all minerals have been removed from it. It also suggests not using softened water for drinking and cooking, since most minerals have been removed from it.

There seems to be no doubt that "hard" water areas have less incidence of heart and circulatory disorders than areas where drinking water is "soft," meaning that it contains fewer minerals. Many scientists have speculated on why this should be. Is it because some minerals in the water actually take part in keeping hearts healthy? Calcium, for example? Or magnesium? Or is it possible that soft water (which tends to leach out minerals) brings toxic minerals like lead and cadmium out of water pipes and this is the reason for the higher incidence of heart problems in these areas? No one is sure of the answer. *The New York Times*, March 7, 1973, reports that the World Health Organization has a group of scientists conducting worldwide surveys to find the answer, if possible.

In their study, WHO scientists in Geneva, Switzerland are clipping toenails and analyzing the metal content of community water supplies, soils and foods as they seek the causes of the rising number of human deaths from heart attacks. The study is one that the WHO is conducting as industrialized countries like the United States and developing countries like Egypt stimulate scientists to solve the mystery of why heart attacks kill so many citizens, especially world leaders like President Lyndon B. Johnson and Egyptian President Gamal Abdel Nasser.

"The scientists are relying on a peaceful use of atomic energy—nuclear activation tests—to detect metals like cadmium, chromium, cobalt, copper, magnesium, nickel and zinc in samples taken from the environments in which men, women and children live in 16 countries in all continents," the *Times* reported.

By using "judicious supplements with trace minerals, vitamins and hormones, a group of physicians from Baltimore, Maryland and Atlanta, Georgia reduced mortality and recurrence of heart attacks in 25 patients whom they treated for six years. There were no new cases of angina (the terrible pain of a heart in distress). None of the patients had to be admitted to hospitals for complications of coronary atherosclerosis—which means obstruction of the important heart artery.

What were other benefits of this simple program involving only trace minerals, vitamins and hormones? All patients found they could exercise more vigorously and for longer periods of time. All circulatory symptoms seemed to taper off during the six-year period. There were no adverse effects. These patients were all earlier victims of severe coronary heart disease. They were doing very badly on the usual heart disease treatment. *Medical Tribune,* August 25, 1971, does not speculate what this program was. Usually it involves several kinds of drugs, including those that "thin the blood"—the anticoagulants. And usually it involves a diet strictly limited as to animal fats—the anti-cholesterol diet. We are not told how strict was the diet on which these patients were maintained. However, we do know that results were far from encouraging.

So the doctors decided to try some trace minerals, vitamins and hormones. They gave their patients the minerals (zinc, copper and manganese), along with "moderate doses of vitamins E and C," and small doses of estrogen and thyroid hormones. Usually, half of the patients with heart conditions as serious as these can be expected to die within five years. Only one patient from this group died, and none of the other 24 suffered a new heart attack. So apparently the diet and hormone program was eminently successful.

"The specific dietary supplements used were chosen on the basis of previous observations of their roles in cellular metabolism and in heart disease," the researchers stated.

It seems impossible that these physicians could have read much in all the extensive material that appears in medical journals (chiefly foreign ones) about the role of vitamin E in the treatment of heart conditions. It seems, too, that they have read little of all the recent discussions about the effectiveness of vitamin C in circulatory conditions, as well as in all-round safeguarding the health of cells and the physiological cement that binds all body cells together. Otherwise, they would surely have given larger doses of these two essential vitamins and perhaps achieved results in a much shorter time.

Speaking of heart attacks, Dr. Stephen M. Ayres, Director of the Cardiopulmonary Laboratory at St. Vincent's Hospital, New York City, stated that the present levels of carbon monoxide in the air "are sufficiently high to represent a major threat to those with coronary disease." He thus urged the Environmental Protection Agency to enact 1975 auto pollution standards on schedule to avert further injury to humans, according to the *New York Post,* March 23, 1973.

"Dr. Ayres noted that patients who have heart attacks when levels of carbon monoxide are high have less chance of surviving than persons who suffer heart attacks on days with low concentrations of carbon monoxide," the *Post* said.

Two Russian scientists report in a 1971 Russian journal that they tested levels of copper, zinc, nickel, manganese and molybdenum in people with various rheumatic diseases. They found unusual levels of zinc and molybdenum in people with acute rheumatic diseases. In chronic inflammatory diseases, the accumulation of most of the trace minerals varied more than in the case of acute disease. No one knows as yet what any of this portends, but it may indicate that the trace minerals play some part in preventing or—if imbalances exist—in causing some of these conditions.

But doesn't it seem possible, you may be asking yourself at this point, that people who would be troubled by excessive amounts of harmful accumulations of trace elements must be only those who actually work in industries where these metals are widespread contaminants? Not at all. As we will state throughout this book, air and water pollution makes all of us—even infants and children—subject to poisoning by whatever pollutants happen to be in air, water and food.

In the *Journal of the American Medical Association* for January 18, 1971, we read the results of a study of the trace mineral content of hair from the heads of 168 fourth grade school children living in five different cities. All these children had lived in their present localities for at least three years.

In City A, which had lead and zinc mining and smelting industries, the boys' hair contained 1.1 part per million (ppm) of arsenic; 2.1 ppm of cadmium; 13 ppm of copper; 52 ppm of lead; 160 ppm of zinc.

In City B, where lead and zinc smelting were the chief industries, concentrations of arsenic in the hair were 4 ppm; cadmium, 1.6 ppm; copper, 12 ppm; lead, 20 ppm; zinc, 145.2 ppm.

In City C, where there was only copper smelting, arsenic levels were 9.1 ppm; cadmium, 1 ppm; copper, 11 ppm; lead, 13 ppm; zinc, 160 ppm.

In City D, which was a center mostly of government and commerce, but which was located near City B, there were 0.7 ppm of arsenic; 0.9 ppm of cadmium; 11 ppm of copper; 7.9 ppm of lead and 160 ppm of zinc in the children's hair.

In City E, where education and farm trading were the chief occupations, arsenic levels were only 0.4 ppm; cadmium only 0.8 ppm; copper 11 ppm; lead 6.5 ppm; and zinc 155 ppm.

Obviously, children growing up in City A are getting almost three times more arsenic from their environment than children in City E. They are also getting almost three times more cadmium, almost 10 times more lead, and somewhat less of copper and zinc. If or when our scientists discover what human disorders may be caused by high accumulations of copper, arsenic and cadmium, how will anyone be likely to associate it with the childhood of children who grew up in certain manufacturing towns? Such detective trails will be impossible to follow, for children, once they are grown, scatter to the four corners of the earth.

The scientist who presented these figures, D. I. Hammer, M.D., of the Ecological Research Branch, Environmental Health Service, Durham, North Carolina, said that the amount of any metal in the hair represents only about half of one per cent of that metal accumulation in the entire body. "The question of increased arsenic and lead burdens and subclinical biochemical abnormalities must be resolved by future investigations," Dr. Hammer said.

In other words, we know almost nothing about the vague, troubling but not seriously disabling or fatal complications that may follow exposure to too much of some of these trace minerals. That is what the word "subclinical" means. Perhaps fatigue, nervousness, restlessness, insomnia, digestive disorders, mental upsets and so on may be such evidence. How many years will it take to untangle all these skeins of relationships and discover whether or not such-and-such a pollutant may bring on such-and-such a condition?

As we have seen, the macro-elements or major elements are present in the body in larger quantities. They are constituents of proteins, cell walls and mechanical structures, like bone, teeth, etc. They play a part, too, in biological activities in the body, but they are mainly occupied with structural things.

The micro-nutrients, or trace minerals, do not have important structural roles, since they are not present in sufficient quantity. Since they are only traces, their role is mainly catalytic—that is, they help to control the physical processes inside our bodies. If they are not present, essential reactions may not take place, resulting in illness or death.

In plants trace elements are present mostly in seeds. In animals they are most abundant in the unborn young.

In the case of laboratory animals confined to cages to be studied, it may take several generations for the supply of a given trace mineral to become exhausted, if it is not given in food. And it is only then that definite symptoms of deficiency will occur. But, as Dr. Karl Schütte points out in *The Biology of Trace Elements,* all such deficiencies are relative. They are usually not due to absolute absence of one or another trace mineral, but rather to deficiencies brought about by altering the ratio among the various elements, resulting in nutritional imbalance. We will see this again and again in our study of the various trace elements.

We have said that trace elements are catalysts. This means that they are used to speed up various happenings inside our bodies, which would take place only very slowly without them. Catalysts can wear out and must be replaced. Dr. Schütte tells us that trace mineral deficiencies have been recognized since earliest times, although not, of course, in terms of modern biochemistry. The Romans knew that anemia was caused by lack of iron, and, having no instant panaceas, they gave anemic people rusty water to drink. Two thousand years ago the Greeks knew that the terrible scourge of goiter could be treated by giving people in a goiterous region the ash of sponges to eat—rich in iodine. In those times, of course, no one had any conception of the infinitely small amount of this trace mineral which was needed to bring about these miraculous cures.

Thus, some minerals are good guys and some are bad guys. As this book progresses, we will discuss each of them in more detail, giving the recommended dietary allowance (if one has been established), and explaining what may happen if you are short on specific minerals. Some minerals, of course, are toxic and we will tell you why.

CHAPTER 4

Tooth Decay May Be Related to Our Mineral-Starved Diets

A SWEDISH BIOLOGIST believes we should attack the problem of tooth decay from the point of view of evolution. Does that seem peculiar to you? What could evolution teach us about the holes in the teeth of today's children?

Alfred Aslander, Ph.D., presented his startling theory in the April-June 1972 issue of the *Pakistan Dental Journal*. Looking back at history and pre-history, we find that human beings came originally from that part of the world which is now East Africa. "If we conclude that evolution will mold each species after its environment we must accept the theory that man, during millions of years of evolution in East Africa, became adapted to conditions prevailing in this part of the world," says Dr. Aslander. "For one thing, it is near the equator in a hot climate. That may explain the adaptation to an almost hairless body."

Our scientists have found bones in that part of the world which are millions of years old, an amazing circumstance, Dr. Aslander explains, because bones disintegrate rapidly in most soils. How then does it happen that here and only here are these very well preserved bones found? He goes on to say that bones are made up chiefly of calcium phosphate and calcium carbonate. Such minerals are easily dissolved in the acids which might be present in the rainfall of a humid, rainy climate.

So, in order for bones to be preserved in soil, the soil must be in a fairly dry climate where rainwater would not percolate frequently through the soil and it must be a location where the soil is so rich in minerals that any water coming in contact with the soil is already saturated with minerals and cannot take up any more. This is exactly the situation in that part of the world, reports Dr. Aslander.

"Our ancestors were thus—for many millions of years— on a mineral-high diet," Dr. Aslander continues. "Evolution adapted man to an environment rich in minerals, providing a mineral-rich nutrition. We may claim: Our ancestors acquired a pronounced need for a good mineral nutrition in order to grow normally, a far better mineral nutrition than civilized man enjoys today. Civilized man is mineral starved."

He points out that animals and plants seek out those places to live where they find conditions like the ones under which they evolved or developed. The American buffalo lived only in the fertile plains where buffalo grass grows. Migrating birds seem to require special habitats for rearing their young, which need vast amounts of certain nutrients to grow into adults.

Those plants which require large amounts of minerals in soil cannot survive in soils less rich in minerals. Oats, for example, can be grown in less fertile soil than barley. Plants preserve, in their cultivated or domesticated state, the same needs they had when they were wild plants. They are, you might say, genetically bound to seek out the kind of surroundings they *must* have, nutritionally speaking.

"For millions of years Nature molded man into a hunter on a savanna in East Africa with the nutritional conditions prevailing there, presumably not only offering a daily food rich in minerals but simply giving no choice, the environment must have been so rich in minerals that all food and all water was rich in minerals," Dr. Aslander says. So our ancestors must have developed over all that space of time requiring rich mineral nutriment. Civilization, as such, is a matter of recent times, in relation to all the millions of years of pre-history.

"Dental caries is commonly described as a bacterial disease," Dr. Aslander adds. "This conception is wrong. The bacteria in cavities is a secondary phenomenon. Dental caries is a deficiency disease. A completely nourished tooth is immune against dental carries. Only starved teeth are attacked by the disease. A tooth is an independent individual that grows out of the mandible (the bone of the lower jaw) in about the same way a plant is growing out of the soil."

In order for a plant to grow, it must have the proper mineral nutriment. So must the tooth. If one or more soil nutrients are lacking, no plant will grow at all. If one or more essential nutrients are not present in adequate amounts, then the plant begins to grow but develops poorly and may show signs of deficiency disease. The same is true of a tooth, says this Swedish scientist. "Complete nutrition produces a strong tooth that will not be attacked by dental caries (that is, decay)".

Tooth decay is somewhat akin to osteoporosis, reports Dr. Aslander. That disorder is the softening process which attacks bones in later life, especially middle-aged and older women who do not eat or absorb enough calcium-rich foods. Mineral deficiency seems to be the leading cause of this bone disorder; the same is true of teeth.

"The food must contain enough of all the minerals needed for the formation of a strong skeleton and healthy teeth," reports Dr. Aslander. "If the mineral supply in the food is insufficient the skeleton will be weak and the teeth begin to decay. That the teeth are especially sensitive toward a faulty mineral nutrition can be explained by the assumption that the teeth contain some rare minerals that are of special importance for a normal metabolism, and the blood takes what is needed where it can be found."

So the need for large amounts of minerals is hereditary in human beings, says Dr. Aslander. He describes the excellent health and legendary longevity of the Hunza people who live in a remote region which has not yet succumbed to "civilization." The land there must be very rich in minerals, he says, and the drinking water which comes from glaciers is so rich in minerals that it has a milky appearance. In present-day Africa, as we know from the writings of many other scientists, when native African people leave their rural communities (where they live on wholly natural food) and migrate into African cities where they eat the "civilized" diet—with its large amounts of white bread, tea and sugar—they soon develop teeth as poor as those of the white men who brought this kind of diet to Africa.

"A healthy diet!" exclaims Dr. Aslander. "Tea is rich in fluorine, which has been vigorously proclaimed to protect the teeth against dental caries. In this severe test, fluorine had no protective effect which is in accordance with our knowledge of tooth nutrition. The fluoridation movement has really very little or nothing to do with dental health, the fluoridation propaganda is strictly commercial. It is an attempt to get rid of a very poisonous and, for the environment, very dangerous industrial waste product by spreading it in a very thin 'layer' over as wide an area as possible."

Dr. Aslander tells us of a study of a remote community in Norway which, for years, could be reached only on skis. Bone eating was common, he notes. The residents ate mutton and lamb, eating the bones along with the meat. They had excellent teeth. Twenty years later a road was built to this community and teeth began to decay as the mineral-poor foods came in to replace the meat and bones. His own parents in Sweden ate bones, says Dr. Aslander, and they had perfect teeth. By the time he was born, they had stopped this practice of bone-eating and his own teeth were less than perfect.

It is possible to produce perfect, decay-resistant teeth by a diet rich in the minerals essential to build strong teeth, Dr. Aslander believes. This kind of diet must start, presumably, in the mother before the child is born, and must prevail from the moment of birth, during the time the teeth are forming and thereafter. We know, he says, that this effort will produce teeth that are immune to decay. We do not yet know whether following this kind of diet will have the effect of improving teeth which have not gotten this good start in life.

"Nutrition of civilized man does not meet the natural requirement (for minerals). Mineral deficiency is common, causing, among other diseases, dental caries. . . . A tooth is primarily a mineral structure; for its formation and maintenance a sufficient mineral nutrient is a pre-requisite. The more we are using unprepared (that is, unprocessed) food, fruit and raw vegetables as our ancestors did, the more minerals we will obtain. . . . Our ancestors were probably bone eaters. And we have every reason to believe that they had perfect teeth."

Dr. Aslander believes that we should all take bone meal as a daily supplement. Bone meal is rich in all essential minerals, its two chief ingredients being calcium and phosphorus. And some researchers think we should, instead, take calcium supplements, for they feel that, if we eat lots of meat and cereal products, we are already getting plenty of phosphorus while we may lack calcium. The relation of these two minerals to one another, as we will find out in later chapters, is important to good health. They should exist in our diets in a certain proportion to one another. And the average modern human diet tends to be-high in phosphorus and low in calcium.

Today we are buffeted on all sides with propaganda about the wonders of fluoridation in preventing tooth decay, with the U. S. Public Health Service and the American Dental Association driving the bandwagon. Once in a while in the medical and dental journals someone suggests that other trace minerals might have the same beneficial effects that are claimed for fluoride, without any of the possibly harmful side effects. No one pays much attention to these suggestions. After all, The Establishment is busy promoting fluoridation.

About 12 years ago some revealing information on tooth decay and diet came from four New Zealand scientists. They incriminated the condition of the soil in which food is grown as a certain contributing cause of tooth decay.

One could not ask for a more clear-cut and obvious experiment than the one described in *Nature* for May 28, 1960; in *Soil Science* for December 1961; and *Nature* for May 5, 1962—all of them written by these investigators. Here is the story they tell.

The public health authorities planned to fluoridate the water in a small New Zealand city—Hastings. Napier, a neighboring city, was to be used as the "control" city (unfluoridated). Before fluoridation was started, a complete dental examination was given to the children of both cities.

The two cities had been chosen because they seemed to be as alike as two cities can be—the same kind of people, the same kind of water supply (artesian wells), the same milk supply. There was practically no fluorine in either water supply. Yet the children of Napier were found to have considerably less tooth decay than those of Hastings. As a matter of fact, some groups of children had as much as 57 per cent less tooth decay than similar groups in Hastings.

Proponents of fluoridation tell us that tooth decay is caused largely by a deficiency of fluorides in the water supply, which they can overcome by putting sodium fluoride into the water. But here were two cities drinking essentially the same water, containing the same amount of fluorides and there was this amazing difference in the amount of tooth decay in the two cities. And 57 per cent less tooth decay in the one city is just about the percentage of reduction in decay the fluoridators claim they can produce by fluoridating water!

The New Zealand scientists believe the explanation lies in something that happened in the city of Napier in 1931. There was an earthquake which raised the lagoon near Napier above sea level, making dry land of it. Citizens gradually moved onto the land which had formerly been the bottom of the lagoon, dug it up for gardens and grew their food there. New Zealanders, it seems, do not generally eat food that has been grown hundreds of miles away and shipped in, as we do. Their truck farms are located near the cities and there are many individual families who raise their own vegetables in their private gardens.

Could the food raised on land from the lagoon be responsible for the difference in the rate of dental decay? The researchers thought it might be. So they tested the vegetables eaten by the residents of both cities—vegetables because these are an excellent source of trace minerals. Sure enough, they found that vegetables eaten by the Napier people (where tooth decay was *low* among children) contained more trace minerals than those eaten in Hastings. Most particularly, the trace mineral molybdenum was found to be more abundant in the Napier food. The scientists thought this might come about due to a difference in the acidity of the soil which had been below the sea for so long.

To check their theory, the scientists decided to feed several groups of laboratory animals on foods raised in the two localities, to see if they could produce tooth decay incidence corresponding to that of the children. They divided their animals into four groups. The first group was fed what laboratory workers call a "cariogenic" diet. This means simply that, other things being equal, this diet will always produce tooth decay in the animals. 68 per cent of this diet is sugar. In addition, it contains vitamins, fats and so on.

The second group received the decay-producing diet, plus the minerals from food grown and eaten in Hastings. The third group ate the decay-producing diet plus minerals from food grown and eaten in Napier. Then, to help decide how much the one trace mineral has to do with it, they fed the fourth group the decay-producing diet, plus the minerals from Hastings food, plus enough molybdenum to make the Hastings food equal to the Napier food in this one element.

Results were most revealing. The animals who received no additional minerals had by far the largest amount of tooth decay. Those eating the minerals from Hastings food had more cavities than those eating minerals from Napier food. The Hastings food to which the trace mineral molybdenum had been added produced fewer cavities than the Hastings minerals alone. *But, this diet was not so good at stopping tooth decay as the diet containing all the Napier minerals.*

The researchers admit that they do not know why this should be. It appears, they say, that it is not just the additional molybdenum in the Napier diet that protects their children from tooth decay. It must be the interaction—the interrelationship—between molybdenum and other trace minerals in the Napier food that makes the difference.

The *Proceedings of the Society for Experimental Biology and Medicine,* Volume 109, 1962, an American scientific journal, reported on the work of investigators at the University of Indiana who found that, by adding both molybdenum and fluorine to the drinking water of the rats in their laboratory, they could get three times the reduction in tooth decay, which they could get by adding just fluorine or molybdenum. This seems to be confirmation of the work done by the New Zealanders.

And both stories seem to point unmistakably to the conclusion every health conscious person came to long ago: the minerals in the soil in which food is grown have a great influence on the health (in this case, tooth health) of the people who eat the food grown on this soil.

Every new thing we learn from nature teaches us that there is nothing isolated in Nature. Things work together in the complex web of life in which all living things exist. To put one trace mineral—fluorine—into the water supply and claim that this is the answer to tooth decay is just as foolishly unscientific as to deny that the presence or absence of trace minerals in the soil in which food is grown has any effect on the health of the people who eat food grown in this soil.

If you are interested in seeing to it that you get plenty of trace minerals in your food, the best idea—which we will mention often in this book—is to raise it yourself, organically if possible. If this is impossible, buy organically grown foods if they are available in your area. In any case, supplement your diet with trace minerals. Kelp is rich in trace minerals.

Processed food contains little or none of this valuable food necessity, so eat fresh, unprocessed foods: raw seeds and nuts, fruits and vegetables, all rich in trace minerals.

CHAPTER 5

There Are Abundant Sea Minerals in Kelp

SCIENTISTS TELL US that the greatly over-populated world of the future may not have enough to eat, unless we turn to the sea and harvest its nutritional riches—fish, shellfish, algae, etc. There is another kind of food that comes from the sea which people have been eating as a staple food in many parts of the world. It's called kelp, a term which applies to any of the large, brown seaweeds belonging to the *Laminariaceae* family. Kelp is dried and powdered for human consumption.

It is believed by scientists that life began in the sea and that the blood which flows in our arteries and veins is a relic of sea water. We know that the composition of blood is very much like that of sea water, so far as minerals are concerned. An editorial in the *Journal of the Medical Society of New Jersey* explained it this way: "The salinity (saltiness) of our body fluid mimics the salinity of the ocean . . . and much of human physiology may be thought of as movement of fluid and electrolytes (minerals) across semi-permeable membranes."

In other words, we are composed of many cells through the walls of which flow salty fluids—blood, lymph, etc. In the healthy person, the various minerals present in this salty fluid are in perfect balance, so that the movement of fluids through the walls of cells is maintained in perfect balance. How can we tell what amounts of the many, many minerals we need to maintain this perfect balance? There is no way of knowing. Although much important scientific work has been done, it may be a very long time until we know everything about trace minerals and what quantities of each of them we need for perfect health.

Meanwhile, we must depend on our food to supply us with minerals. We know that we can get calcium from milk and milk products; iron from meat and eggs; phosphorus from seeds; etc. But what about the trace minerals? Of course, calcium, phosphorus and potassium are supplied when commercial fertilizers are applied to the soil. But what about vanadium, boron, bismuth, manganese, copper? One answer is kelp.

Extracts from seaweeds such as Irish moss, kelp and rockweed find more than 40 different uses in the food, drug, textile and farming businesses. From several provinces of Canada more than $1 million worth of seaweed is harvested annually. Yet we actually know little about this product. Fortunately, more and more scientists are studying it. As they do, they are finding that it appears to be something of a wonder-substance.

A group of Canadian scientists have been working on seaweed extract—sodium alginate—as protection against radioactive strontium, that substance which causes so much concern since it is related to atomic explosions and thereafter contaminates our food for many years. In carefully controlled and designed experiments, these Montreal researchers gave rather large amounts of the extract to laboratory rats at the same time that they gave them measured amounts of radioactive strontium in their food. They found that the seaweed extract kept the animals from absorbing the harmful strontium. It bound the mineral in such a way that it passed out of the body without damage.

How this knowledge can be used to protect human beings is the next question to be solved. There seems to be no evidence that adding the extract to all our diets would do much to protect the general public from the radioactivity that is still in much of our food, as a result of those early bomb tests (and the few tests that are still being done), but it does seem likely that the seaweed extract can be used in case of some grave emergency or accident where radioactivity heavily contaminates the food supply of a group of people.

In such an eventuality they can be given the extract in large amounts, almost like a medicine, and possibly be protected from any permanent damage. This is, therefore, a valuable piece of information to have in these days when atomic reactors are springing up like mushrooms almost everywhere and radioactive materials are being used in an increasing number of industrial and medical operations. The Canadian experiments were reported in the *Canadian Medical Association Journal* in 1964.

A Chicago physican found in 1965, and reported in the *Annals of the New York Academy of Science*, that a

Mineral Content of Sea Kelp

Element	Percentage by Volume	Element	Percentage by Volume
Aluminium	1.00	Iodine	0.15
Strontium	0.10	Cobalt	0.001
Nickel	0.10	Manganese	0.100
Chromium	0.05	Iron	1.000
Barium	0.005	Copper	0.100
Titanium	0.005	Potassium	12.49
Gallium	0.005	Magnesium	0.72
Bismuth	0.004	Calcium	2.76
Tin	0.004	Phosphorus	0.32
Vanadium	0.001	Sodium	15.04
Silver	Trace	Sulfur	1.04
Molybdenum	Trace	Silicon	1.00
Zirconium	Trace	Boron	0.005
Zinc	0.003		

material extracted from crude kelp was capable of killing viruses which cause influenza. Studying the action of the material, Dr. Ralph H. Kathan found that it seemed to surround the virus and thus prevent its entrance into a cell. Such an experiment does not seem to give us any practical help in fighting off germs at present, but it certainly points the way to a future in which harmless, healthful materials like kelp may be solving our problems with germs, rather than the quite hazardous antibiotics we are using now.

At an International Seaweed Symposium, held in 1965, two Norwegian scientists reported on the use of seaweed supplements in the raising of cattle and pigs. Here is something which we can apply to everyday living. It is well known that the sea contains rich stores of minerals. As more and more soil erodes and is washed into the sea, its mineral supply increases. Obviously, plants growing in the sea take up these minerals as they grow. Can we use such minerals as a source of the trace minerals that are so necessary for good health?

Drs. Harold Nebb and Arne Jensen fed dairy cows on a mixture of fortified seaweed meal and compared the results with another group of cows being fed on a commercial mineral mixture. The seaweed meal was found to be equal in every way to the commercial one and, indeed, led to greater milk production. In feeding pigs, the seaweed also proved quite as effective as a commercial mixture of minerals. The experimenters added calcium, phosphorus and vitamin D to the seaweed, since these are not present in seaweed in significant amounts. Seaweed does contain vitamin A, vitamin E, some B vitamins, iodine, zinc and potassium, in addition to many trace elements. Kelp, on the other hand, contains over 26 trace minerals, such as barium, boron, chromium, gallium, nickel, silicon, silver, strontium, titanium, vanadium, sulfur, copper, sodium, etc.

Kelp's content of the minerals that exist in larger

amounts is quite astonishing. It contains almost two-tenths of one per cent of iodine, compared to clams (another rich source) which contain only 1,900 parts per billion. Kelp has one per cent iron and more than 12 per cent potassium. Compare this to the potassium content of almonds (a rich source) which have only 0.7 per cent of this mineral. By using powdered kelp to replace iodized salt, you would get almost 10 times more iodine than you get from the commercially prepared salt.

In many parts of the world, different kinds of kelp or seaweed are used for food, just as we use salad greens. In parts of Japan seaweed makes up a large part of daily diet. It is significant that goiter is unknown in these communities and it seems certain that the iodine content of the kelp is the reason for this. While iodine given by itself prevents goiter, the dosage must be carefully regulated, for an overdose is dangerous. But we can be sure that we will not get too much iodine in kelp, for it occurs in extremely small quantities in perfect balance with all the other trace minerals that are present.

Is kelp palatable? Many people enjoy eating it flattened into paper-thin sheets. Others do not like the taste, so the most popular way is to sprinkle the "sea salt" on their food, to take it in tablets, or to buy it in various forms available at your health food store. Nutritionists have found that some minerals given in tablet form are difficult or impossible for the human body to assimilate. Iron, for instance, given for anemia, must be in a certain chemical form or it may not be used by the body. Presumably the same is true with other minerals. But minerals in a completely natural form, as in kelp, are well absorbed.

Thus, kelp provides us with an excellent, inexpensive source of trace minerals. Just a few tablets every day will provide at least some of all the trace minerals that make this such a valuable food supplement. You don't need as much of the trace minerals as you do of, say, calcium. So small amounts—sprinkled on your food instead of salt, for example—are quite valuable.

There is one warning about kelp. If you are on an absolutely salt-free diet, you will have to remember that kelp contains considerable sodium—the substance you are trying to avoid. But such diets are rare. Many of us have been told to cut down on salt. This we can do easily by using kelp as a salt substitute. Since it contains so many more minerals than plain salt, its sodium content is only about one-tenth that of table salt. Why not consider adding this valuable food as a supplement, especially if your family is reluctant to eat fish and seafoods, which are our only reliable source of the important mineral iodine.

CHAPTER 6

Calcium

CALCIUM IS THE most abundant mineral in the body, comprising 1.5 to 2.0 per cent of the weight of an adult's body, report Milicent L. Hathaway and Ruth M. Leverton in *Food,* the U.S. Department of Agriculture Yearbook for 1959. Calcium is usually associated with phosphorus, which is 0.8 to 1.1 per cent of the body weight. A person who weighs 154 pounds would have 2.3 to 3.1 pounds of calcium and 1.2 to 1.7 pounds of phosphorus in his body.

About 99 per cent of the calcium and 80 to 90 per cent of the phosphorus are in the bones and teeth, according to *Food.* The rest is in the soft tissues and body fluids and is highly important to their normal functioning.

"The human embryo," *Food* continues, "at 12 weeks contains about 0.2 gram of calcium and 0.1 gram of phosphorus. (There are 28.4 grams in an ounce). The values are 5.5 and 3.4 grams, respectively, for the two minerals by the 28th week, and 11 and 7 grams by the 34th week. The most rapid increase in the calcium and phosphorus content of the unborn child occurs from the 34th week to the 40th week.

"One-half of the total calcium and more than one-third of the total phosphorus in the baby's body at birth are deposited during the last six weeks. The baby's body contains about 23 grams of calcium and 13 grams of phosphorus at birth.

"The calcium content of the body," *Food* says, "increases faster in relation to size during the first year of life than at any other time. About 60 grams of calcium are added. A child is depositing only about 20 grams a year when he is 4 or 5 years old and weighs about 40 pounds. He may be depositing as much as 90 grams a year when he is 13 to 14 years old and weighs 110 pounds. He will deposit more if he weighs more. All these gains in calcium depend on an adequate supply of calcium in the diet and the ability of the body to use it for normal growth."

In addition to providing strong bones and teeth, calcium prevents rickets in children. It helps to prevent osteoporosis or softening of the bones in older folks. It is essential for normal clotting of the blood. It nourishes nerve tissues and its deficiency results in cramps and, in extreme cases, convulsions. And it helps the heart to maintain its normal beat. Its functions, incidentally, are closely related to those of magnesium, phosphorus, sodium and potassium.

Physicians have known for some time that people confined to bed for long periods of time lose calcium in their urine during this period of bed rest. This is one reason for the modern practice of getting patients out of bed as soon as possible after operations or other therapeutic emergencies. The longer they stay in bed, the harder it is for them to recover normal function after they do get up. There are many reasons for this. One of these is undoubtedly just that they have lost so much calcium from bones and blood.

Doctors have said, "Well, we'll increase the amount of calcium they get and thus lick the problem." Or they have said, "We'll make them exercise while they are still in bed and the exercise will correct this tendency." Now new research has uncovered the fact that neither of these two expedients will have any beneficial effect. You lose calcium when you are lying on your back for long periods of time. The only thing that will correct this and return

How Much Does Calcium Cost You?

Milk Product	Market Unit	Portion providing as much calcium as 1 cup fluid milk	Cost of calcium equivalent
Whole, fluid milk	½ gallon	1 cup	$0.07
Nonfat dry milk	12 qt.	1 cup reconstituted (⅓ cup dry milk)	0.03
Evaporated milk	large can	½ cup	0.05
Fresh skim milk	½ gallon	1 cup	0.07
Parmesan cheese grated	8 oz.	⅝ oz.	0.07
Buttermilk	1 qt.	1 cup	0.08
Cheddar cheese, natural	1 lb.	1⅓ oz.	0.09
Ice milk	¼ gallon	1½ cup	0.12
Cottage cheese, creamed	2 lb.	10¾ oz.	0.21
Yogurt, plain	8 oz.	9½ oz. (1 cup)	0.30
Blue cheese, natural	4 oz.	3¼ oz.	0.38
Yogurt, fruit flavored	8 oz.	1⅓ cup	0.40
Coffee cream	1 cup	1¼ cup	0.42
Cream cheese	8 oz.	17 oz.	0.68

the body to a normal calcium balance is standing up.

A physician in a Philadelphia hospital experimented with a number of healthy young volunteers. They were kept in bed lying on their backs for considerable lengths of time. They lost large amounts of calcium in their urine. They were given vigorous exercises which they could take lying on their backs. This did not change the calcium picture. They were given different amounts of calcium in their diet. This did not change the calcium excretion. The bed exercises were increased up to three or four hours daily. There was no effect.

But as soon as the young men were gotten out of bed and required to stand quietly for two or three hours daily, their calcium balance returned to normal. The doctor in charge concluded that it is the action of gravity, rather than anything else, which keeps us from losing calcium when we are spending some of our time standing. This finding would seem to be extremely important for many groups of people. First, the astronauts have been having difficulty with this problem. It seems likely now that equipment will be redesigned to change their position in their capsules. What the astronaut medical team will do to provide gravity in an environment where there is no gravity is anybody's guess.

As for the rest of us, it seems important to realize that anyone in our family who is steadily confined to bed for any reason is going to be better off, so far as calcium is concerned, if he can be gotten to his feet for several hours a day. This does not mean sitting in a chair, but standing, even if it means constructing elaborate devices for propping him up if he is unable to stand by himself. Walking is preferable, if this is possible, since this will benefit feet and legs and general circulation.

At the opposite end of the pole, we have a report from Eastern Europe that extreme physical exertion increases calcium excretion. According to three researchers in a Romanian journal, human beings who were fed plenty of calcium, phosphorus and protein, then given several weeks of intense daily muscular activity, were found to be in what is called "negative calcium balance." When the amount of calcium they ate was increased to almost twice what it had been, they once again became normal.

So in this case, it seems that increasing the calcium in one's diet will help immeasurably if one is planning to saw wood, or go deep sea diving or run races or something of the sort. Even a day of shopping or mowing the lawn or cleaning the basement might be a less nerve-wracking experience if you take an extra glass of milk to provide the extra calcium necessary. Of course, it will provide extra protein as well.

Today our nutrition specialists believe they know most of the functions of calcium in our bodies. And the one thing that everyone is agreed on is that you can't get along without this mineral. In fact, you can't get along very well if you are even a bit deficient in it. How many times have you heard middle-aged people say they never drink milk because milk is a food for children. "Children must have the calcium of milk for forming bones and teeth," they agree. "But you don't need much calcium as you grow older." How wrong such sentiments are and what nutritional trouble they can get you into is constantly being spelled out in the medical journals.

On February 23, 1968, the U. S. Department of Agriculture released a survey indicating that 20% of the families surveyed had poor dietary habits. One of the nutrients most often found in short supply was calcium. For example, the survey discovered that 31 per cent of the families in the Northeast; 31 per cent in the North Central; 30 per cent in the South; and 31 per cent in the West were short on calcium. Those surveyed were from all economic strata, not just lower-income families.

In an article in the March 1955 issue of *Iowa Farm Service*, Dr. Pearl Swanson of the Iowa Agricultural Experiment Station and a collaborator from the U. S. Department of Agriculture reported on "You Don't Outgrow Your Need for Calcium." They describe a survey made

---

Calcium Content of Foods

Almonds	234 milligrams in ¼ pound
Bread, whole wheat made with dried milk	118 milligrams in 3 slices
Buttermilk	121 milligrams in ½ cup
Carob flour	352 milligrams in ¼ pound
Cheese, cheddar	750 milligrams in ¼ pound
Cottage	94 milligrams in ¼ pound
Swiss	925 milligrams in ¼ pound
Collards	250 milligrams in ¼ pound
Dandelion greens	187 milligrams in ¼ pound
Filberts	209 milligrams in ¼ pound
Kale	249 milligrams in ¼ pound
Milk, whole	590 milligrams in 2 cups
Powdered, skim	1,308 milligrams in ¼ pound
Mustard greens	183 milligrams in ¼ pound
Sesame seed	1,600 milligrams in ¼ pound
Seaweed, kelp	1,093 milligrams in ¼ pound
Soybean flour, defatted	265 milligrams in ¼ pound
Whey, dried	646 milligrams in ¼ pound
Yogurt	590 milligrams in 2 cups

---

among more than 1,000 Iowa women to discover how much calcium they were getting in their daily meals. All the women were 30 years old or older. They were a representative cross-section of the population, so they actually represent about half a million Iowa women who eat as they do.

The experts who conducted the survey found that only one woman in every five was getting in her meals and snacks the amount of calcium recommended officially as the best amount. The reason was simple. They didn't drink enough milk or use enough foods that contain milk —cheese, yogurt, etc. Although they were eating fairly good diets from the point of view of other nutrients, their supply of calcium was so low that they could expect, as time went on, to be bothered by many kinds of disorders that result from lack of calcium.

"Middle-aged bones seem to break more easily than young ones," says Dr. Swanson, "and we think this occurs largely because calcium has been withdrawn and not replaced. Our hip bones, for instance, carry much of the body weight. If the calcium in our diets is inadequate, the hip bones may become so weak that they are no longer able to support this weight. Thus, a bone may break and we fall. We usually think that a person falls and breaks a bone. But physicians tell us that very often the bone breaks first and causes the fall."

What did the Iowa women eat that gave them fairly adequate supplies of other nutrients, but not enough calcium? Here is a list of a typical day's menu. It includes: a serving of meat, fish or poultry, an egg, several slices of bread, a serving of white potatoes, a serving of corn, an orange or some orange juice, a serving of tomatoes and one of peaches, a salad of lettuce, cucumbers, radishes and onions, a little cream, some butter and salad dressing, a piece of cake, some sugar and jelly. Does this sound like the kind of food most of your family and friends eat?

Well, such a diet contains about 300 milligrams of calcium. The recommended daily allowance of calcium is 800 milligrams for an adult—more than twice what these women got in their daily food. For the record, the RDA for girls from 11 to 18 years of age is 1,200 milligrams of calcium. "Such a diet cannot be regarded as satisfactory," says Dr. Swanson.

By adding two cups of milk, these women could bring their daily calcium intake up to the recommended amount. The milk, of course, can be taken as a beverage, used in cooking, or eaten in various forms. One ounce of cheddar cheese supplies about as much calcium as ¾ cup of milk.

About one-third of American women over 50 suffer from osteoporosis. This is a condition, as we have stated, in which the bones "thin out" and become weak. The spine and pelvis are the two regions most often affected. There is some scientific evidence that osteoporosis is caused chiefly by lack of the sex hormones, which the body no longer manufactures during and after middle age. Hence, some doctors prescribe hormones to prevent or treat osteoporosis. But such treatment is fraught with dangers. It is expensive for one thing. It does not cure any basic condition, but merely continues to postpone indefinitely a perfectly natural process. And it frequently has many unpleasant side effects.

A number of recent scientific and medical journals have reported that diet can and will prevent and treat osteoporosis. Bones are composed of an organic framework made mostly of protein, and of calcium which is deposited in the protein structure. In the normal adult, old bone is continually being reabsorbed and new bone must be manufactured. This is a normal part of life and the essential building materials must be provided or this process cannot go on normally.

Note the presence of protein in bones. They are not just plain mineral. To maintain bone protein, we must have enough protein at meals or in food supplements.

Protein is found chiefly in foods of animal origin—meat, fish, poultry, eggs, dairy products. Vegetarians get their protein chiefly from soybeans and other seed foods like nuts and whole grain cereals, as well as brewers yeast and wheat germ. The officially recommended daily amount of protein, as announced in 1974 by the National Academy of Sciences, is 52-56 grams for men and 46-48 grams for women.

Some researchers now believe that older folks may have the same need for vitamin D that babies have. Since many of the oldsters do not spend much time outdoors in the sunshine, perhaps they should be taking supplements of vitamin D, since this vitamin is almost completely absent from food. An exception, of course, is milk, which has, normally, 400 USP units of vitamin D added per quart. The Recommended Dietary Allowance for vitamin D is 400 units. Two French scientists, writing in *Presse Medical*, November 9, 1963, state that one of the major causes of osteoporosis may be lack of vitamin D.

A British Columbia physician, writing in the *Canadian Medical Association Journal* for January 23, 1965, states: "Vitamin D must be present to ensure adequate absorption of calcium." He suggests no more than 400 units of vitamin D daily.

Writing in the *Journal of the American Geriatrics Society*, June 1962, Dr. M. L. Riccitelli said: "Osteoporosis in the aged is probably due to a combination of poor nutrition, loss of . . . sex hormones and inactivity or immobilization. In old people deficiencies of protein, vitamins and calcium may result from anorexia (lack of appetite), certain food habits, unbalanced diets, lack of teeth, food idiosyncrasies, serious and prolonged illnesses or economic conditions . . . there is a tendency toward low blood levels of thiamine (vitamin B1), ascorbic acid (vitamin C), carotene (vitamin A) and other vitamins despite adequate intake, absorption and assimilation of these substances . . . (this) may be due to either an hepa-

How Much Calcium Do You Need?

According to the National Academy of Sciences, we need calcium every day in the following amounts. We give the amounts in milligrams (or mgs).

Men and women need . . . .   800 mgs.
Pregnant and lactating women need . . 1,200 mgs.
Infants need . . . . 360-540 mgs.
Children 1-10 years old need . . . .   800 mgs.
Boys 11-18 need . . . . 1,200 mgs.
Girls 11-18 need . . . . 1,200 mgs.

tic dysfunction (liver trouble) . . . or an increase in the physiologic need for vitamins beyond the requirements for adults and children."

"In individuals accustomed to low calcium intakes, osteoporosis is more common than in those who have had higher dietary intakes of this mineral . . . requirements of amounts of dietary calcium . . . increase with age in both men and women . . . Shorr and Carter were able to produce significant storage of calcium in some patients with osteoporosis by raising dietary calcium intake to 2 grams or more daily," reports *Osteoporosis, a Disorder of Mineral Nutrition*, by Leo Lutwak and G. Donald Whedon.

States J. L. Newman in *Journal of the New Zealand Dietetic Association*, December 1962: "It is now believed that bone formation is not defective in persons with osteoporosis but that there is a calcium deficit. Special attention should be given to . . . patients' diets, both by insuring plenty of foods with a natural calcium content and also by the addition of mineral calcium to them (that is, food supplements)."

"There are increasing data to suggest that in both sexes as good if not better results can be achieved with a high supplementary calcium intake as with steroids (sex hormones)," reports Hamish W. MacIntosh, M.D., in the *Canadian Medical Association Journal,* January 23, 1965. "The use of calcium is simpler, cheaper and less hazardous. A calcium supplement of 3 grams daily should be given. One gram of calcium is provided by 4 one-gram tablets of di-basic calcium phosphate. Eleven one-gram tablets of calcium gluconate or 13 half-gram tablets of calcium lactate will provide the same amount of calcium."

"Many patients with these forms of osteoporosis absorb and retain calcium abnormally avidly when on a high calcium intake in the form of supplements and moreover may continue to retain it avidly for at least three and a half years. Symptoms of the disease are relieved and no further fractures take place," says *Lancet,* volume 1, 1961, page 1015.

"Calcium salts, in doses of 2 to 3 grams daily, have been shown to induce a positive calcium balance . . . serum (blood) vitamin D levels in osteoporotic patients are below normal . . . some bone biopsies have demonstrated changes which might be the result of a relative vitamin D deficiency; and . . . vitamin D administration has resulted in increased calcium retention," says the *Journal of the American Medical Association,* May 18, 1964.

An excellent leaflet, *Facts About Osteoporosis,* is available from the Information Office, National Institute of Arthritis and Metabolic Diseases, Public Health Service, Bethesda, Maryland.

If you are taking calcium supplements, it might be wise to take the calcium at night, just before retiring, rather than during the day. This is the theme of an article in the *British Medical Journal* for June 2, 1973. Four physicians from the London Hospital in England tell us that it seems most calcium is lost from bones during the night, in cases of osteoporosis. Apparently the calcium that you may take with meals is absorbed within three hours after you take it. So by midnight any effect of the evening meal in raising calcium levels of the blood would have ceased.

In women past the menopause it seems that calcium is needed to suppress the action of a certain hormone which tends to cause bones to soften. If most of the blood calcium is gone before retiring, therefore, the hormone could perform its debilitating work during sleep. Doctors have found that, before the menopause, women excrete much less calcium in the morning than women who are past menopause. This seems to indicate that something, overnight, causes the body to lose calcium—presumably from bones—in the woman who has passed menopause.

The London doctors did tests on a group of 49 women, giving some of them a supplement of calcium (800 milligrams in all), which they took just before going to bed. They were told to eat as usual during the day and, of course, to include foods with a lot of calcium. Then the doctors checked the amount of calcium excreted in urine during the night and immediately upon rising. They found that less was excreted when the calcium supplement was taken just before retiring. So they suggest that women past the menopause who are trying to prevent osteoporosis should take calcium supplements in one dose, just before going to bed, rather than extending it, in smaller doses, throughout the day.

They're finding rickets in school children in Birmingham, England, according to Dr. William T. Cooke of the Birmingham General Hospital. Cases of deformed bones severe enough to be detected on X-ray have been found in about 5 per cent of 600 children at five Birmingham schools. Twenty per cent of those affected had both clinical and biochemical evidence of the disease. Cases are also turning up in London and Glasgow.

Rickets, as we know, is a disease of deficiency of calcium and vitamin D chiefly. The calcium must come from milk and other dairy products. The vitamin D can come only from sunshine, which is very scarce in the

British Isles in winter. Vitamin D, of course, can be given by irradiating milk to produce vitamin D in the milk; or it can be given in supplements.

It seems a peculiar turn of events, when England announces a minor epidemic of this easily prevented disease from lack of vitamin D probably, that our own Food and Drug Administration has decreed a reduction in the amount of vitamin D allowed in food supplements. Perhaps we can look forward to an epidemic of rickets in our own country, since the FDA has succeeded in curtailing the vitamin D we have been getting.

Dangers in migration from southern to northern climates are pointed out in an article in *Lancet* for April 28, 1973. Six Scots physicians studied rickets and osteomalacia in immigrants from Asia to Britain. Osteomalacia

Minerals and Trace Minerals in 100 Grams of Milk

(About ½ cup of liquid milk or cottage cheese)

Minerals	milligrams
Calcium	118
Iron	0.057
Magnesium	13
Phosphorus	93
Potassium	144
Sodium	50

Trace minerals	micrograms
Aluminum	350
Boron	60
Bromine	400
Chromium	1.4
Cobalt	0.13
Copper	32
Fluorine	30
Iodine	35
Manganese	5.5
Molybdenum	6
Nickel	6.5
Selenium	2.5
Silicon	82
Vanadium	Trace
Zinc	450

is a bone-softening process in older people caused by a deficiency in calcium, phosphorus and/or vitamin D. There is, of course, much less sunlight in Britain than in the southern parts of Asia. Compared with the level of a similar group of Northern Europeans, the Asians had far less vitamin D in their blood. Those who had symptoms of either deficiency disease had less vitamin D than those who appeared to be without symptoms.

Say the physicians, "It seems that vitamin D deficiency is the major factor leading to rickets and osteomalacia in Indian and Pakistani immigrants to Britain."

It should be noted that, some time back, officials in Scotland decided to cut down on the enrichment of milk and other foods with vitamin D. Cases of rickets, as we have just noted, have been increasing since then. In the older people studied by the Scots physicians, the bone softening process seems to occur because so many of them are house-bound and never get out into the sunshine. The researchers theorize that there may be a large, undiscovered number of such victims.

Dr. John M. Ellis, in his book, *Vitamin B6, the Doctor's Report*, tells of treating 225 cases of pregnancy complications with pyridoxine (vitamin B6). He says that leg cramps in pregnant women can persist, even though they are taking calcium. The cramps disappear when pyridoxine is added to the calcium, he adds.

A Swiss scientist, reporting in the Swiss medical journal, *Schweizerische Medizinische Wochenschrift* (April 1, 1967), has found that quite large amounts of calcium taken at mealtime lead to a significant lowering of the cholesterol levels of blood in the 20 patients who were observed for four weeks. He gave them more than 1½ grams of calcium daily at meals. In addition to lowering the cholesterol levels, the calcium also lowered levels of other fatty substances in the blood. When he injected calcium, there was no effect on these levels. It had to be taken by mouth.

MINERALS: KILL OR CURE?

Dr. Carl J. Reich of Calgary, Alberta, Canada, wrote to the *Canadian Medical Association Journal* (August 29, 1972), as follows: "I believe that mineral deficiency is more common in people today than is usually suspected. As a means of correcting this deficiency, I would like to suggest that for people who do not consume two glasses of milk or two ounces of cheese a day, small sealed envelopes containing sterilized bone meal should be made available with fresh or processed meat. Instructions on the envelope could indicate how the bone meal might be used, at the rate of 1 gram per pound of meat, to dust the meat before cooking or to be added to gravy or vegetable sauce." Bone meal, we might add, is a rich source of minerals, including calcium.

According to an abstract in *Clinical Medicine* for May 1969, calcium is what you may need for healthy fingernails. Dr. T. James states that nobody knows exactly why it is that fingernails break. Taking gelatin every day (the unsweetened, health food store kind) for quite long periods has been suggested, since gelatin is almost entirely protein. But now it appears that calcium plus some vitamin D—to make sure you absorb the calcium—may help the gelatin.

A Cornell University professor of psychiatry has discovered that the body's use of calcium is upset by various curative procedures used by psychiatrists. He studied patients in a mental hospital, all of whom were getting the same amount of calcium in their diets and all of whom were being treated with electric shock or a tranquilizer. He discovered that some of the patients with certain kinds of mental disorders lost calcium in their urine consistently during treatment. Those with other disorders did not. And, significantly, the patients who continued to lose calcium during the treatment were those who improved. The ones who did not improve did not show a difference in the way their bodies used calcium.

The professor asks if it might be possible that the loss of calcium had something to do with the patients' ability and opportunity to move around. And he came to the conclusion that, because of the excellent therapy being given these particular patients, their mobility or lack of it could not have influenced the results. So he concludes that calcium is certainly involved very closely in the improvement or lack of improvement of patients with certain kinds of mental illness.

In the April 2, 1971 issue of the *Washington Post*, there is the pathetic story of how many patients in Maryland mental institutions were suffering from pellagra (the vitamin B3 or niacin deficiency disease). Dr. Neil Solomon, a specialist in nutrition, visited the hospital kitchens and studied the menus. He found that the meals were deficient not only in niacin, but also in protein, iron and calcium.

"Diet and nutrition play an important role not only in caries (decay) production, but also in the rate of degeneration of the bone and gingiva (gums) supporting the teeth," says Dr. Harry Roth, a New York periodonist, in *Drug Trade News* for May 27, 1963. "Vitamin A, the B Complex, vitamin C, vitamin D, calcium, phosphorus and protein are needed for repair of alveolar bone, connecting tissue and epithelium which comprise the periodontium. These nutrients are woefully lacking in many of the patients' diets."

Thus, we have seen that calcium plays an important role in human nutrition. It makes for strong bones and teeth; it is essential for the clotting of blood, the action of certain enzymes, and the control of the passage of fluids through the cell walls. And the right proportion of calcium in the blood, states *Food*, is responsible for the alternate contraction and relaxation of the heart muscle. Additionally, the irritability of the nerves is increased when the amount of calcium in the blood is below normal.

We should, therefore, manage to get a full two cups of milk or its equivalent every day. You can't substitute anything else for calcium. And without milk it is almost impossible to get the recommended daily amount. Can't you get calcium from fresh leafy vegetables? Yes, but you must eat large amounts of these every day. For instance, you would have to eat three pounds of cabbage or two pounds of endive, or one pound of cooked kale, or two pounds of lettuce or one pound of mustard greens to get the 800 milligrams of calcium in 2 cups of milk. In addition, there is the problem of absorption. Some leafy vegetables contain substances that make the absorption of calcium difficult. But milk digests and is absorbed perfectly in all normal, healthy people.

Yogurt and goat milk, cup for cup, contain the same amount of calcium as cow's milk. In addition, yogurt contains the helpful lactobacillus bacteria which are good for digestion and the health of the digestive track. Shop for yogurt at your health food store and try to get a brand that does not contain a lot of hidden sugar. The best idea, of course, is to buy a yogurt maker at the health food store and make your own yogurt at home.

Goat milk has the added advantage of being naturally homogenized. That is, the fat and non-fat parts of the milk are naturally mixed in such a way that they do not separate as they do in cow's milk. Some people find this milk much easier to digest because of this natural homogenization. Also, goats are generally raised by health conscious people who have small dairies and take great pains to feed and care for their animals. So you are likely to get goat milk that has come from the healthiest possible animals, which have never been exposed to pesticides or all the many drugs and additives that are common in the food of animals at most large dairies.

And don't forget cheese. In a booklet, *Cheese Varieties*, the U.S. Department of Agriculture tells us that the making of cheese goes back to very ancient times. No one knows who made the first cheese, but the story goes that an Arabian merchant in olden times put some milk into a pouch made of sheep's stomach and started on a journey across the desert. The rennet (an enzyme in the lining of the pouch) converted the milk into cheese and whey. The merchant liked the taste of the cheese and slaked his thirst with the liquid whey.

Until the middle of the 19th century, cheese was strictly a local farm industry. Housewives made it at home from milk that was not used for drinking. The first cheese factory in the United States was built in 1851. Since then, cheese has become largely an industry product. At present more than a billion pounds are made each year in the U.S., with about one-tenth of our milk being used for cheese.

The USDA booklet goes on to name more than 400 varieties of cheese, grouped under four headings: very hard cheeses used largely for grating (Parmesan and

---

Nutritive content of 100 grams of cheese
(This means about ½ cup cottage cheese, or ¼ pound of harder cheese.)

Protein _____
  17-36 grams

Fat _____
  0.3 to 37.7 grams

Carbohydrate _____
  1.6 to 2.9 grams

Calcium _____
  62 to 1140 milligrams

Phosphorus _____
  95 to 781 milligrams

Potassium _____
  72 to 149 milligrams

Vitamin A _____
  10 to 1240 International units

Thiamine _____
  0.01 to 0.08 milligrams

Riboflavin _____
  0.25 to 0.75 milligrams

Niacin _____
  0.1 to 1.2 milligrams

Romano); the hard, like cheddar, swiss and gruyere; the semi-soft (Munster, Limburger and Roquefort); and the soft, such as cottage, ricotta and cream cheese.

Cheese contains large amounts of protein and calcium. It is one of our richest sources of the B vitamin riboflavin (vitamin B2), which is extremely scarce in other foods. Cheese has almost no carbohydrate and may contain as much as 37 per cent fat (in cream cheese).

If you are trying to avoid saturated fats (those from animal sources), cottage cheese should be your choice for there is only about one-third of one per cent of fat in uncreamed cottage cheese. The creamed kind is only 4.2 per cent. Cottage cheese is 13-17 per cent protein, meaning that you get almost 20 grams of good, high-quality protein in one-half cup of cottage cheese.

For some reason, many restaurants list cottage cheese as a vegetable. If you are trying to keep weight down, order it, rather than other "vegetables," such as sweetened applesauce, sherbet or carbohydrate-high lima beans or potatoes. Aside from this, you should choose your cheese mostly on the basis of what you like. Many of them contain lots of sodium, so if you are on a low-sodium or low-salt diet, choose the ones that seem to be less salty, or, better still, ask your health food store about low-salt cheese. And try to avoid those cheeses that contain a lot of additives. There are dozens of worthwhile cookbooks that will tell you how to use cheese.

There are other excellent sources of calcium available at your health food store. Sesame seed with hulls, alone among all the seed products, is quite rich in calcium. One-fourth of a pound contains more than 1,000 milligrams of the mineral. And, of course, there are many calcium food supplements available.

If you are allergic to milk or for some reason cannot use it, the calcium supplement becomes an absolute essential. And even if you do use lots of milk, the added calcium in a supplement will be beneficial. There is little danger of your getting too much calcium if the rest of your diet is well balanced.

No doubt some of you have wondered why some manufacturers offer phosphorus-free supplements while others stress the fact that their product contains both phosphorus and calcium. In most American diets there is plenty of phosphorus and probably not enough calcium. Of course, we don't know what your diet consists of, so we are getting into that familiar trap of referring to the well-balanced diet. But, to put it simply, if you are one of those Americans who get lots and lots of phosphorus in your daily diet but are probably not getting enough calcium, then you will probably want to take a supplement of calcium which contains no phosphorus. Presumably you are already getting enough phosphorus—right? If, on the other hand, you make a real effort to get plenty of the high-calcium foods every day and feel certain you are getting enough calcium, then you may wish to take a mineral supplement which contains both these minerals, along with iron, magnesium, copper, etc.

Why not check through your daily diet and that of your family, for a week or so, just to make certain everyone is getting enough calcium. Pay special attention to the very young and the very old family members. They need lots of calcium and they may not be getting it. Refer to the charts for the amount of calcium in various foods, as well as the recommended amount of calcium for various age groups.

CHAPTER 7

Phosphorus

PHOSPHORUS AND CALCIUM are of equal importance in the bones, according to *Food*, the Yearbook of Agriculture, 1959. Phosphorus is involved in ossification or calcification of bone just as much as calcium. When bone is formed, phosphorus is deposited with the calcium. When the bone loses calcium (by decalcification), it also loses phosphorus. They are also closely associated in blood and foods. Phosphorus is included, therefore, even though it is not named each time that calcium is mentioned.

"The intricate process of bone building requires many nutrients besides calcium and phosphorus," *Food* states. "Vitamin D is essential for absorption from the intestinal tract and the orderly deposition of the bone material. Protein is needed for the framework and for part of every cell and circulating fluid. Vitamin A aids in the deposition of the minerals. Vitamin C is required for the cementing material between the cells and the firmness of the walls of the blood vessels.

"Bones can accumulate a reserve supply of calcium and phosphorus at any age if the diet provides enough for the growth and repair and some is left over for storage," *Food* continues.

"When the intake is generous, the minerals are stored inside the ends of the bones in long, needlelike crystals, called trabeculae. This reserve can be used in times of stress to meet the body's increased calcium needs if the food does not supply enough.

"When there is no reserve to use, the calcium has to be taken from the bone structure itself—usually first from the spine and pelvic bones. The dentin and enamel of the teeth do not give up their calcium when the body must provide what the diet lacks.

"If the calcium that is withdrawn in times of increased need is not replaced," *Food* notes, "the bone becomes deficient in calcium and subnormal in composition. From 10 to 40 per cent of the normal amount of calcium may be withdrawn from mature bone before the deficiency will show on an X-ray film. Height may be reduced as much as 2 inches because of fractures of the vertebrae, which are caused by pressure and result in rounding of the back. Such fractures may occur with relatively minor jolts or twists of the body and may not be recognized at the time they happen."

The Yearbook points out that a low content of calcium in the bones makes them weaker and thus they break more easily than bones well stocked with calcium. Breaks, especially in older people, often are related directly to the thinness and brittleness of the bones and are difficult to treat. The bones may be too weak to hold pins or other means of internal repair, and healing may be slow because of the low activity of bone-forming cells.

"The calcium and phosphorus and other minerals in our food are dissolved as the food is digested. Then they are absorbed from the gastrointestinal tract into the blood stream," *Food* says. "The blood carries them to the different parts of the body where they are used for growth and upkeep.

"Calcium as it is present in food dissolves best in an acid solution. It begins to dissolve in the gastric juice of the stomach. The calcium is absorbed when the contents of the stomach move into the small intestine. Farther along in the intestine," we are told, "the contents change from an acid to alkaline reaction, which does not favor the absorption of calcium."

It is estimated that 10 to 50 per cent of the calcium eaten is not absorbed but is excreted in the feces. A small portion of the excreted calcium comes from the intestinal fluids.

"The calcium that is absorbed travels in the blood to places where it is needed, particularly the bones. If any of the absorbed calcium is not needed, it is excreted by the kidneys into the urine. Normal functioning of the kidneys is essential for the normal metabolism of calcium and other minerals," according to *Food*.

Phosphorus performs more functions than any other mineral in the body. As we have stated, it combines with calcium to create healthy, strong bones and teeth. It occurs in body fluids, in every cell of the body and it is an essential part of just about everything that goes on there. It helps in the working of muscles; it helps the body to break down fat, carbohydrate and protein into body structures; it is involved with the health of nerves and blood. It is partly responsible for transporting fatty substances in the body.

Phosphorus, like calcium, is absorbed most effectively when the strongly acid digestive juices are present in the stomach and intestines. As we grow older, these digestive juices tend to decrease, so the older person may actually need more phosphorus (and calcium) than the younger person, just because he may absorb less from his food. So the older person who shuns seeds and nuts, meat and eggs may lack phosphorus. If he also dislikes milk, he is almost certain to be courting a calcium deficiency. In the United States, 70 to 75 per cent of the calcium in our diets comes from milk and other dairy products; 15 to 20 per cent from plant foods; about 5 per cent from meat and eggs; and some from water and the compounds con-

taining calcium that are used in commercial food processing, reports *Food*.

Television commercials for antacids are rampant. You are urged almost incessantly to stop that acid trouble in your digestive tract by taking such-and-such a pill or powder. In 1968, three National Health Institute scientists showed that prolonged taking of antacids produces deficiency in phosphorus. They tested six patients with prolonged antacid treatment and discovered that they developed too little phosphorus in the blood and in the urine, increased absorption of calcium in the stomach, finally too much calcium, increased draining of calcium and phosphorus from bones, which produced lack of appetite, weakness, bone pain and malaise (body weakness or discomfort, which often means the onset of a disease). The antacid used was magnesium aluminum hydroxide, and this experiment was reported in the *New England Journal of Medicine* for February 22, 1968. And, according to *Food*, laxatives also are likely to lower the absorption of calcium.

"A hormone secreted by the parathyroid glands has an important part in the body's use of calcium and an indirect part in the use of phosphorus," states *Food*. "There are two of these tiny glands on each side of the neck near or in the thyroid gland. The parathyroid hormone keeps the amount of calcium in the blood at a normal level of about 10 mg. per 100 milliliters of blood serum. (Serum is the watery part of the blood that separates from a clot.)

"Any wide deviation from this amount is dangerous to health and life," continues *Food*. "The hormone can shift calcium and phosphorus from the bone into the blood. If the blood levels are too high, it can increase the excretion of these minerals by the kidneys. If anything reduces the secretion of the parathyroid hormone, the calcium in the blood drops quickly, the phosphorus rises, and severe muscular twitchings result.

"The amount of calcium absorbed into the body is affected by the body's need for it, the amount supplied by the diet, the kind of food that supplies it, and the speed with which the food passes through the gastrointestinal tract," *Food* says.

The Yearbook reports that lactose—the form of sugar present in milk— is especially good in promoting the absorption of calcium. Certain proteins and amino acids are also effective. It is believed that the combination of these is responsible for the excellent absorption of calcium from milk.

But the absorption of calcium from vegetables is somewhat lower. The high content of fiber, especially in the coarse, leafy, green vegetables, makes them move through the intestine rapidly, and the amount of calcium absorbed is somewhat reduced.

Foods Rich in Phosphorus

(The figures are given in term of one average serving —about ¼ pound)

Food	Milligrams of Phosphorus	Food	Milligrams of Phosphorus
Almonds	504	Pumpkin seed	1,144
Beans, kidney	406	Rice bran	1,386
Beans, mung	340	Rice polish	1,106
Beef	200	Safflower seed	
Bran flakes	495	meal	620
Chicken	265	Sesame seeds	616
Chickpeas	331	Soybeans	554
Cowpeas	426	Soybean flour,	
Eggs, 2	200	defatted	655
Filberts	337	Sunflower seed	837
Flounder	344	Sunflower seed	
Lentils	377	flour	898
Liver	476	Wheat bran	1,276
Peanuts	407	Wheat germ	1,118
Peanut flour	720	Yeast, brewer's,	
Pine nuts	500	1 tablespoon	945

"Spinach, beet greens, chard and rhubarb contain a chemical—oxalic acid—which combines with the calcium to make calcium oxalate. Because it is insoluble in the intestinal fluids, the calcium cannot be absorbed but is excreted in the feces," *Food* says.

"The outer husks of cereal seeds, such as wheat, contain phytic acid, a substance that combines with phosphorus to form phytates. The phytates can interfere with the absorption of calcium, especially in a child when a high intake of phytic acid is accompanied by an inadequate supply of calcium and vitamin D."

Phytates are not likely to hinder the absorption of calcium, iron, zinc, magnesium, etc., in the diets commonly used in the United States. But unleavened bread—that is, bread made in the Eastern way using no yeast or baking powder—is not very healthful from the point of view of nutrients absorbed. This bread is popular with some of the young people who favor natural foods.

Dr. John G. Reinhold of the Pennsylvania Nutrition Research Project in Iran studied different kinds of bread sold in Iran and the results on the people who ate these breads. His survey was concerned mostly with the phytate content of the bread. Phytate exists in cereals and is especially abundant in wholegrain flours. That is, it accompanies that part of the flour which is removed during refining.

In some villages of Iran, Dr. Reinhold found that bread constitutes up to 75 per cent of the total diet. Some of this was unleavened; it was made of wheat and water and baked in thin loaves with no fermentation such as occurs when yeast is added. Sure enough, Dr. Reinhold found that some of the Iranians were suffering from zinc deficiency, although there was apparently enough of it in their diets. In those places where bakers made the bread and raised it with yeast, no mineral deficiencies were noted.

Writing in *Ecology of Food and Nutrition,* 1972, Vol. 1,

pages 187-192, Dr. Reinhold concluded by saying that, when bread makes up the largest part of the diet, it should be leavened. If wholegrain bread is eaten without being leavened, it is likely to cause loss of minerals to such an extent that it could be injurious to health.

As we know, meat, fish, eggs, dairy products, cereals and nuts are all rich in phosphorus. These foods make up a considerable part of our meals, so it is unlikely that any of us lack phosphorus. But all of these foods—except milk —tend to be rather low in calcium. And that is where the difficulty arises. These two minerals are inexorably linked in such a way that you cannot neglect one and expect the other to be used by the body to perform all the functions it is supposed to perform.

Let's say you plan to eat the very best possible diet, from the point of view of protein and vitamins . . . and even food supplements. You eat lots of meat, fish and poultry. You add wheat germ and brewers yeast, excellent sources of B vitamins and minerals. You eat eggs and nuts for their protein, their vitamins and their wholesome fats. But, for one reason or another, you decide not to add any milk or dairy products. You have designed a diet rich in almost every food element . . . *except calcium.*

Such a diet, because of its high phosphorus content, makes your need for calcium even greater. So, although you are eating all these nourishing foods, you might end disastrously and suffer very seriously from disorders involving calcium deficiency. Leafy vegetables contain considerable amounts of calcium relative to other foods, but, even if you added these to the diet outlined above, it would be extremely hard to eat enough of them to balance the large amounts of phosphorus in the meat-cereal-seed-egg-rich diet.

There seems to be a sound nutritional reason why "bread and cheese," "bread and milk," or "oatmeal and milk" are established partners in diet in many parts of the world. Mexicans who live mostly on tortillas made from ground corn (rich in phosphorus) add limestone (rich in calcium) to the corn when they grind it. Centuries of observation have shown these people who have certainly never studied nutrition that they need a source of lime or calcium when they eat large amounts of cereal or seed foods. Refer to the chart for the phosphorus and calcium content of some common foods. As you see, there are very few in which the calcium content comes anywhere near the phosphorus content.

Wheat germ contains, gram for gram, more phosphorus than any other food except brewers yeast and not a great deal of calcium, relatively speaking. Does this mean that you should not eat wheat germ or brewers yeast? Not at all. It means that you should be careful to include plenty of calcium in your meals at all times. If you love wheat germ (and we hope you do), if you eat a lot of it and add it to many other foods to enrich them, or if you are eating large amounts of brewers yeast, then you need more calcium to balance the phosphorus you are getting.

Sesame seeds and sunflower seeds are extremely rich in phosphorus. Dry soybeans contain more phosphorus than meat. Since soybeans are the nearest thing to a vegetarian complete protein food, it is not surprising to find that they are also a rich source of calcium. Soybean flour is unmatched as a source of both calcium and phosphorus. Powdered milk contains about 13 times as much calcium as wheat germ, so you would do well to add powdered milk to foods containing wheat germ or brewers yeast and eat plenty of milk when you use wheat germ as a breakfast cereal. Cheese is another food rich in phosphorus and calcium, thus an excellent addition to any meal.

And don't forget that all nuts are good sources of phosphorus. We recommend eating them without salt or roasting, just as they come from the shell. And don't forget that other delicious snack food—seeds. All are rich in phosphorus, as well as protein, healthful fats and iron.

Look for both seeds and nuts in your health food store.

How much phosphorus do you need? The Recommended Daily Dietary Allowances, as revised in 1974 by the Food and Nutrition Board, National Academy of Sciences, are:

	Mg.
Infants	
To five months	240
5 months to 1 year	400
Children	
1 to 3	800
4 to 6	800
7 to 10	800
Males	
11 to 14	1,200
15 to 18	1,200
19 to 22	800
23 to 50	800
50 and over	800
Females	Mg.
11 to 14	1,200
15 to 18	1,200
19 to 22	800
23 to 50	800
50 and over	800
Pregnant	1,200
Lactating	1,200

CHAPTER 8

Iodine

ACCORDING TO *Food for Us All*, Yearbook of Agriculture, 1969, a man who weighs around 160 pounds may be made up of about 100 pounds of water, 29 pounds of protein, 25 pounds of fat, 5 pounds of minerals, 1 pound of carbohydrate and one-quarter ounce of vitamins. As we know from previous chapters, most of the mineral material is calcium and phosphorus, found deposited in the protein framework of bone and tooth cells to create a hard tissue able to bear weight and pressure. There are, of course, numerous other minerals and trace minerals present. One of these is iodine.

"By 1930, as newer techniques and apparatus made it possible for chemists to measure minute amounts of certain inorganic substances," reports *Food*, "the significance of the trace elements in nutrition was recognized. Iodine had been identified a century earlier. In the 1920's it was identified as an essential nutrient. The thyroid gland at the base of the neck enlarges when it is deprived of iodine.

"The condition is known as simple goiter. In the Great Lakes area, where iodine has been leached out of the soil and so is not available in food or drinking water, goiter used to be a common occurrence among children, especially girls."

One of the earliest large-scale controlled human experiments was conducted by David Marine and O. P. Kimball in 1921 with six thousand school children in

Akron, Ohio, *Food* reports. They showed that children given iodine in drinking water did not develop goiter; a large proportion of those not so treated did develop this condition. A more effective way of providing a readily available and safe supply of iodine for all people was developed later by adding potassium iodide to table salt. Use of this salt has always been on a voluntary basis, but it provides a wise public health measure available to all people, *Food* adds.

So for many centuries no one knew what caused the horrible symptoms which were noticed most often among mountain people and those who lived far from the sea. Most of the people had swollen throats and bulging eyes. Children might be born dwarfed, mentally retarded, with rough skin, sparse hair, brittle nails and a tendency toward constipation, anemia and a distinctive, awkward way of walking.

Even after modern science discovered that all these disabilities resulted from lack of a single trace mineral— iodine—it was almost impossible for people to believe that lack of a single substance—just a tiny amount of a single substance—could produce such ravages in the form of poor health. But whenever this precaution is ignored, even in inland parts of our own country, goiters begin to appear again and all the troubles of iodine deficiency become manifest.

"Iodine is an essential nutrient for man, its sole recognized function in the human organism is its role in the formation of thyroid hormone, of which it is a basic component," according to the *Heinz Handbook of Nutrition*, a valuable reference compiled by leading authorities on nutrition.

The thyroid gland, which uses most of the iodine in our bodies, manufactures the substance, or hormone, thyroxin, which is responsible for bringing about many activities in the body. Perhaps most important, the thyroid gland, through its hormone, regulates the rate at which our bodies burn the food we eat. This is called the "basic metabolic rate," that is, the rate at which the resting human body uses oxygen in the combustion of carbohydrates, protein, fat and other food substances. You can see from this that iodine is extremely important for good health. This has been known for thousands of years.

In ancient days, doctors used to burn sponges from the sea and give the ashes to people with disorders of the thyroid gland, such as goiter. They did not know why the ashes improved the condition. Now we know that sponges, along with other products of the sea, are loaded with iodine. The iodine was present in the ashes.

For many years, people in various parts of the world have suffered from goiter and other disorders of the thyroid gland because their soil lacked iodine. So the food grown there lacked iodine. The thyroid gland, deprived of enough iodine, grows large in an effort to compensate for this lack. In areas where there is plenty of iodine in the soil, and in areas close to the sea and in individuals who habitually eat seafood of all kinds, goiter and other disorders of the thyroid gland are practically unknown. In Japan, for example, where seaweed is considered a gourmet dish and is eaten every day, goiter is unknown. In other Far Eastern countries where diet and the way of life are much like the Japanese, but seafood is not eaten, goiter is common.

The use of iodized salt has done much to improve the world situation in regard to goiter. Where this enriched salt is used, apparently enough iodine is obtained for good health, even though sea foods, fish and seaweed are not eaten. But many people do not use iodized salt, for one reason or another. People placed on salt-poor diets are likely to lack iodine unless they get it from some other source.

According to *Nutrition Research* for July-August 1955, iodine-rich dried seaweed or kelp would provide about

10 times more iodine if it were used as a condiment instead of iodized salt. In iodized salt the iodine preparation is added to plain sodium chloride, or table salt. On the other hand, kelp, being a completely natural product, contains many other vitamins and minerals in addition to its iodine—magnesium, potassium, calcium, iron, copper, sulfur, etc.

An expert on seaweed in the diet, Dr. W. A. P. Black of the British Nutrition Society, says, "It can be said that seaweed contains all the elements that have so far been shown to play an important part in the physiological processes of man. In a balanced diet, therefore, they would appear to be an excellent mineral supplement."

Recent investigations have shown that perhaps man is in danger of getting too much iodine from his environment—that is, from various kinds of man-made pollution and chemicalization. We have, for example, noted the high iodine content of baker's bread containing dough conditioners.

Dr. W. T. London of the National Institutes of Health discussed at a "Trace Element" symposium in 1964 the occurrence of iodine as an air and water pollutant. He found that the vegetation growing in a median strip of a well-traveled highway contained much more iodine than vegetation away from the highway. He found also that the purification treatment of water is adding iodine to our rivers and streams. Sewage plants are adding iodine to river water in a concentration about 40 per cent of that found in sea water.

Dr. Hans T. Shacklette of the U. S. Geological Survey has found that animals and human beings absorb iodine from the atmosphere where it is present. An article in the *Canadian Medical Association Journal* for March 9, 1963 relates the story of a group of Tasmanian children who were given a potassium iodide food supplement to prevent goiter. At about the same time the school lunch program began to provide free milk for all the children. Soon it was found that in some areas the incidence of goiter had increased rather than decreased. It was then that public health authorities found that the cows whose milk was sent to the areas where goiter was increasing had been fed almost exclusively on kale. This is a member of a family of foods (including cabbage) which, if eaten exclusively, interfere with the uptake of iodine by the thyroid gland.

"It is important to remember," says the *U. S. Department of Agriculture Handbook for 1959*, "that life is a delicate balance of a seemingly infinite number of competing chemical and physiological processes."

Oysters are an excellent source of iodine. They are also rich in protein (about 9 grams in ¼-lb. of cooked oysters), iron (8 mg. per serving), vitamin A and the entire B Complex. Oysters and other shellfish answer the need for iodine, and they are readily available—fresh, frozen or canned.

The Recommended Daily Dietary Allowances, Revised 1974, for iodine are:

Infants (to five months)	35 micrograms
Infants (5 months to 1 year)	45 micrograms
Children (1 to 3 years)	60 micrograms
Children (4 to 6 years)	80 micrograms
Children (7 to 10 years)	110 micrograms
Males (11 to 14 years)	130 micrograms
Males (15 to 18 years)	150 micrograms
Males (19 to 22 years)	140 micrograms
Males (23 to 50 years)	130 micrograms
Males (51 and over)	110 micrograms
Females (11 to 18 years)	115 micrograms
Females (19 to 50 years)	100 micrograms
Females (51 and over)	80 micrograms
Pregnant females	125 micrograms
Lactating females	150 micrograms

CHAPTER 9

Iron

AT LEAST ONE-FIFTH of the world's population lacks iron in their diets, hence in their blood, according to a report delivered to the World Health Organization. *Medical Tribune* for June 7, 1972 tells us that a normal healthy adult should have some 500 milligrams of iron stored in his or her body. But in two studies in Canada and the United States, the younger women were found to have not much more than one-half that level.

Twenty per cent of all American families eat diets that are classified as "poor" by United States Department of Agriculture nutrition experts, according to a survey released on February 23, 1968. Only one-half of all families had what was described as a "good" diet. For iron alone, the USDA survey found that 11 per cent of the diets were deficient in the Northeast; 10 per cent in the North Central; 9 per cent each in the South and West.

In 1969, a Public Health Survey of 12,000 Americans revealed that one-third of all children had iron deficiency anemia. Fifteen per cent of everyone examined (adults and children alike) had iron deficiency anemia. In the richest, best-fed nation in all history, these facts seem unbelievable, but they are true. It is reasonable to suppose that those 12,000 are representative of the rest of the nation, rich and poor alike.

Highlights of the Ten-State Nutrition Survey, a booklet recapping this 1968-1970 Public Health survey, reveals similar deficiencies. "Among the various age groups surveyed, adolescents between the ages of 10 and 16 years had the highest prevalence of unsatisfactory nutritional status. Male adolescents had more evidence of malnutrition than females. Elderly persons were another age group with evidence of increased nutritional deficiencies. Persons over 60 years of age showed evidence of general undernutrition which was not restricted to the very poor or to any single ethnic group. . . .

"There was evidence that many persons made poor food choices that led to inadequate diets and to poor use of the money available for food," the survey states. "In particular many households seldom used foods rich in vitamin A. Also there was a heavy emphasis on meat in many diets, rather than use of less expensive but excellent protein sources such as fish and poultry, or legumes and nuts. Many diets were also deficient in iron content, but this was less a reflection of poor choice of foods than of the generally low level of iron in the American diet. . . ."

Iron is a mineral, rather plentiful in some foods, but very scarce in others, which is essential for the formation of the red pigment that colors our red blood cells. These are the cells which carry oxygen to every cell of our bodies. And they cannot live without oxygen. If they are getting too little oxygen, the function of all these cells suffers. So lack of iron can cause a wide variety of symptoms, from fatigue to inability to concentrate, from paleness to lack of muscle tone.

Indirectly, all organs can be harmed by the lack of oxygen brought about by anemia: heart, lungs, brain, kidneys, digestive tract. Anemic infants may become cranky and irritable. Anemic mothers may be unable to carry on household chores. Anemic adolescents may fail in their school work.

Infants, menstruating and pregnant women and old folks are those most likely to suffer from iron deficiency anemia. Infants are born with only a small store of iron in their bodies. This must be reinforced by food. Since a baby's diet consists mostly of milk, and since milk does not contain a great deal of iron, there is a good chance that children who live mostly on milk for their first year or even longer will not get enough iron to prevent anemia. This is the reason why the wise mother feeds her baby egg yolk, vegetables and whole grain cereals—all rich in iron.

Women may lose a considerable amount of iron in the menstrual flow without knowing their flow is excessive, hence not consulting a doctor about it. Since anemia may predispose one to loss of excessive menstrual blood, clearing up the condition will also prevent its recurrence.

Iron Content of Some Common Foods High in Iron

Food	Milligrams of Iron in an Average Serving
Almonds, ½ cup	3.3
Beans, dried	4.6
Beans, lima	5.6
Beef	3.
Blackstrap molasses, 1 tbsp.	2.3
Chicken	1.4
Clams	6
Collards, cooked	3
Dandelion greens	5.6
Eggs	1.1
Heart, beef	5.9
Liver, beef	4.4
Mushrooms	2
Mustard Greens	4.1
Oysters, 1 cup	13.2
Peas	3
Pecans	2.6
Pork	2.2
Prunes, 1 cup	4.5
Raisins, 1 cup	5.6
Shrimp	2.6
Spinach	3.6
Walnuts, 1 cup	7.6
Wheat germ, 1 cup	5.5

Chronic infections can take their toll of the body's iron at any age. Infected teeth or tonsils, gums or ears that are neglected may produce a quite unsuspected case of anemia. Getting rid of the infection clears up the anemia and prevents its recurrence. However, it may take some time for you to recover from a prolonged bout with an infection which has produced anemia. The body's stores of iron can be rebuilt only slowly. If anemia is the result of internal bleeding, then a careful medical examination and diagnosis are in order. Bleeding ulcers have been known to cause anemia.

In older folks, more easily susceptible to a wide variety of disorders, anemia is prevalent. Some cases undoubtedly arise because of rigid eating habits which are difficult to change. Someone who just doesn't like eggs or meat may find it very difficult to get enough iron at meals unless very careful attention is paid to planning menus and allowing for plenty of green, leafy vegetables, whole grain cereals, nuts, beans and other seed foods. If vegetables are difficult to chew they can be puréed or mashed. Nuts and seeds can be finely ground.

Often overlooked in our thinking about getting enough iron is the fact that certain other food elements are necessary for iron to be absorbed during the process of digestion. Copper is essential—in very small amounts, true. But it is essential. So is vitamin C. If you are eating the recommended all-round good diet, you will, of course, be getting enough of both of these, for copper is abundant in nuts and seeds, shellfish, liver and whole grains. And vitamin C is present in fresh fruits and vegetables. But if someone in your family just can't stand liver and can't be bothered to eat fresh fruits and vegetables, he or she is running the risk of iron deficiency anemia, even though there's plenty of meat and eggs in the diet. There just isn't enough of the other things that are required to digest and use iron healthfully.

"Until recently there has been relatively little information systematically establishing the prevalence of anemia in non-hospitalized American populations," says an article in the *Journal of the American Medical Association* for March 22, 1971. The authors grant that Dr. Arnold Schaefer of the Public Health Service (the 10-state survey that we just mentioned) has turned up some astonishingly grim evidence in this area. They go on to discuss a survey which they conducted in a community in Florida. They took blood from more than 3,000 children to determine how many were anemic. They found, they tell us, that 14.8 per cent of all the infants examined were anemic. Among those who were just approaching their teens, only 2.6 per cent were anemic. However, with increasing needs for iron among teenage girls due to menstruation, it was not surprising to find that the incidence of anemia went up sharply in teenage girls. Among teenage girls who were pregnant, nearly 25 per cent were anemic. "The poor diet often consumed by teenagers may have further aggravated this situation," say the authors.

In the February 5, 1968 issue of the *Journal of the American Medical Association,* an official committee on the AMA's Council on Foods and Nutrition sets forth its findings which show very clearly that there is lack of iron in "a large segment of the female population," that no one knows precisely, if at all, how much iron "the average American" gets in his food, how much he absorbs and consequently how much more he needs.

The facts were gleaned from studies which are hairraising in their implications. One survey showed that 66 of 114 young women had no iron stores, or very little, in their bodies. In another survey, it was found that iron stores were completely absent in 9 out of 13 women studied. In another study, 84 per cent of all women studied had no iron stores in their bodies. What about school children? Well, one study of supposedly normal children showed an incidence of iron deficiency anemia in from 8 per cent to 64 per cent! A study of a group of infants produced the shocking information that half of them were suffering from iron deficiency.

The *Journal* study notes that menstruation, pregnancy and various forms of ill-health all deplete iron stores. In addition, the *Journal* suggests that donating blood is responsible for a loss of 250 milligrams of iron with every donation of 500 milliliters of blood. To replace this loss over a year's time, one would have to increase one's intake of iron by 0.7 milligrams a day. We do not know of any group which accepts blood donations giving out any information on the necessity of replacing the iron lost—do you?

It is well known that not all the iron in food is absorbed. Individuals vary greatly in the amount of iron they absorb from any given food. It is estimated that about 5 to 10 per cent of iron is usually absorbed. People who are deficient in iron may absorb as much as 15 per cent. It is noteworthy, too, that the iron from vegetable food is not as readily or completely absorbed as that from food of animal origin. A serving of spinach may contain 2.2 milligrams of iron, which may not be absorbed as well as the 3.5 milligrams of iron in a serving of beef.

"In recent years, great concern has been expressed about the food habits of the adolescent. Information on the nutritional status and dietary intake of adolescent girls, whether pregnant or not, is limited, although studies on their food habits suggest that they have the poorest dietary habits of any age group," say two Department of Agriculture scientists in the November 1972 issue of the *Journal of the American Dietetic Association*. They go on to tell us that, by 1962, the mothers of 19 per cent of all babies born in this country were 19 years old or younger and that all complications of pregnancy were most prevalent in this group of mothers. Studies done in 1969 showed that there are an alarming number of pregnancies in girls 15 and younger. Along with this disturbing information we now have the news that teenage girls are very likely to be deficient in both iron and folic acid (a B vitamin).

The two researchers decided to find out what they could do about the incidence of deficiency in 114 pregnant girls from 12 to 17 years old who came to a University of Alabama Medical Center. Their status in regard to these two nutrients was compared to that of 40 non-pregnant girls in the same age group. The object was to see how the groups compared in relation to the supposed "requirement" of adolescents for various nutrients.

The researchers are well aware of the shallowness of this kind of survey, for they say, "The term 'requirement' is not easily defined, and nutritional requirement tends to be most descriptive when used for large groups, since some persons' requirements are less than the average and some are more, because of size, activity, sex, pregnancy and lactation. Requirements for a single nutrient are more difficult to define, not only because there may be several levels of nutritional status to which they could be applied, but because of the interrelationships of nutrients. Therefore, it is concluded that the minimum requirements would prevent the clinical manifestations of the deficiency, whereas more of a nutrient would be needed to meet periods of stress, such as pregnancy."

The results of a 3-day survey of the diets of both groups of girls uncovered the fact that neither the pregnant nor the non-pregnant girls were getting anywhere near the amount of iron they need for good health. Where folic acid is concerned, both groups were far below the recommended levels. Since requirements for folic acid are especially high in pregnancy, the pregnant girls were in more perilous condition than the non-pregnant ones. While all of them were risking a very serious kind of anemia which can be fatal, due to lack of folic acid, they were also risking plain iron deficiency anemia as well.

The figures also show that the diets of both groups of girls contained considerably less than recommended amounts of vitamin A, calcium and some of the B vitamins.

"One might have thought," says an editorial in the *Canadian Medical Journal*, February 10, 1962, "that iron-deficiency anemia was not a common condition in a highly developed country like Britain, but two recent papers draw attention to the fact that it is still one of the commonest diseases the general practitioner has to deal with, and that a number of cases do not receive the simple treatment they require."

The physician they quote reveals that in his practice of 5,000 patients, he found a total incidence of 17.5 cases of anemia in every 1,000 patients. There were four times as many women as men; most of them had no other disease, and most of them were severely anemic requiring long treatment with iron medication.

A later article in the *Canadian Medical Journal* (May 12, 1962) tells us there are four important aspects of the way the body uses its store of iron:

1. Normally we lose very little iron by excretion.

2. The body has a very effective mechanism for saving iron that has been used and using it over again.

3. Many things about us influence the absorption of iron from our digestive tracts.

4. "There is a delicate and precarious state of iron balance in most individuals, particularly at certain periods of life, rendering them highly susceptible to development of iron deficiency anemia."

As we know, even though iron is used in relatively small quantities it performs an extremely important function in the body: it is a part of the complex system that carries oxygen to every cell of the body. Hence, it is essential for each individual cell to breathe. Hemoglobin, a substance in the blood containing iron, combines with oxygen in the lungs and releases the oxygen in the tissues wherever it is required. The red blood cells, or corpuscles, in which the hemoglobin is carried in the blood, have an average life span of about 120 days, after which they are destroyed. The iron is salvaged and used to manufacture new, young red blood cells.

Vitamin C is that peculiar substance which human beings must get in their food, although most animals can manufacture it inside their bodies, hence do not need it in food. Vitamin C has many functions in human beings, among them nurturing the small blood vessels, the teeth, bones and skin, preventing hemorrhages, helping in the manufacture of the physiological cement that holds cells together, healing wounds, fighting germs, carrying hydrogen to body cells. In addition to these, vitamin C has a relationship to the mineral iron. The vitamin helps in the absorption of iron through the intestine walls. It would seem, then, if you have some orange juice for breakfast, this will help you to absorb healthfully the iron in your eggs, cereal or whole grain toast.

The British Journal of Nutrition, Vol. 21, No. 2, 1967, carried an article by three Indian scientists who had been working with laboratory rats made deficient in iron. The rat makes its own vitamin C inside its body. It does not have to get it in food. The scientists found that the perennially anemic rats, short on iron, had higher concentrations of vitamin C in their tissues, as well as in their urine. This seems to suggest, they think, that lack of iron raises your needs for vitamin C. That is, the less iron in your diet, the more vitamin C you may need. In the case of the rats, they were apparently manufacturing larger amounts of vitamin C than healthy rats, to make up for the shortage of iron in their bodies. Since human beings cannot make vitamin C for themselves, this suggests that those of us who tend to be anemic from lack of iron should be getting larger amounts of vitamin C than other people.

Another experiment reported in the *Canadian Medical*

Association Journal for July 22, 1967, demonstrated that at least one form of iron is absorbed much more effectively in the presence of quite large amounts of vitamin C. These scientists gave healthy, non-anemic volunteers ferrous sulfate, a medicinal form of iron. Along with it they gave one group of people 50 milligrams of vitamin C and another group 1,000 milligrams of vitamin C. Then they measured the amount of iron in the blood. They found that 50 milligrams of vitamin C did not raise the levels of iron in the blood. But 1,000 milligrams did. So it appears, in human beings, quite a considerable amount of vitamin C may be necessary for the proper assimilation and use of iron.

For years a battle raged over the proposal by the Food and Drug Administration that bread be fortified with iron preparations which would raise its iron content to 45 milligrams in a one-pound loaf. Some members of the medical profession have been opposed to this proposal. On the other side of the scientific scrimmage are many nutritionists, including Dr. Jean Mayer, President Nixon's official nutrition expert, who believes that iron deficiency anemia is so common, especially among pregnant and menstruat-

Table of Nutrient Levels Per Pound

	Enriched Flour New Levels	Old Levels
Thiamine	2.9 mg	2.0 - 2.5 mg
Riboflavin	1.8 mg	1.2 - 1.5 mg
Niacin	24 mg	16 - 20 mg
Iron	40 mg	13 - 16.5 mg

	Enriched Bread New Levels	Old Levels
Thiamine	1.8 mg	1.1 - 1.8 mg
Riboflavin	1.1 mg	0.7 - 1.6 mg
Niacin	15 mg	10 - 15 mg
Iron	25 mg	8 - 12.5 mg

ing women as well as children, that additional iron fortification of bread must be accomplished.

Dr. Philip Lanzkowsky, Professor of Pediatrics at Downstate Medical Center in New York, says in *Medical World News* for September 25, 1970 that so many children are deficient in iron that milk should be enriched with iron. Dr. Lanzkowsky points out that there is plenty of evidence that lack of iron in the diets of infants and children leads to *pica*—that is, dirt-eating of one kind or another. Apparently the child is so hungry for minerals that he eats anything containing minerals. In big cities where old tenements have walls from which the crumbling lead paint has fallen, this childhood appetite results in lead poisoning, which is becoming an epidemic among the urban children.

Giving the child enough iron stops the urge to nibble on the lead-containing paint chips and cures the lead poisoning. Says Dr. Lanzkowsky, "One must question why the condition (of iron deficiency anemia) revealed in numerous surveys over the past 50 years, has been tolerated in a country where well-baby clinics are freely available—particularly when the deficiency is easy to diagnose and cure." He has asked state and federal health officials to frame legislation which would make fortification of milk with iron mandatory.

The National Academy of Sciences-National Research Council estimates that there may be as many as 250,000 women in the United States at any given time who are suffering from iron deficiency anemia. A Northwestern University professor of home economics tells us that surveys demonstrate that the amount of iron women are getting from their food is much less than the official Recommended Daily Allowance.

On the other hand, there is strong opposition to the proposed enrichment program among experts who are equally well-informed and apparently equally objective in their thinking. What it all boils down to is a difference of opinion in regard to what should be done, when considerable segments of the population show up deficient in one nutrient or another.

The health seeker would, of course, suggest that everyone, young and old, get their iron first-hand, from foods which have not been devitalized. In the case of iron this would mean eating lots of whole-grain flours, cereals and bread, wheat germ, bran, whole eggs, meat, liver, leafy green vegetables which make up altogether the best diet anyone can eat, with some dairy products for calcium, and fruit for vitamin C. If everyone in the country were aware of the necessity for eating healthfully and had enough money to buy these foods every day, it seems obvious that the problem would disappear. Trying to solve it by "enriching" those foods which have first been "impoverished" by the milling and baking industries is just not the way to reach a solution.

Dr. Margaret A. Krikker, a general practitioner of Albany, New York, has made a study of supermarket foods to which iron has been added. She says that many foods are already fortified and that, if the amount of iron in bread is increased, some people will be getting too much. She mentions the disease hemochromatosis, which is known as the "iron-storage disease." No one knows what causes it. It is believed to be genetic—that is, the person is born with an unnatural ability to store too much iron. There is increased iron in the blood, in the liver. The disease can be fatal. (It seems obvious that victims of this disease could easily be put on special diets which would not include foods enriched with iron!)

Dr. William H. Crosby, Jr., chief of hematology at New England Medical Center Hospital, is quoted in *Medical World News* for January 21, 1972 as saying, "You have these two disease groups: millions of women with iron deficiency and tens of thousands of men with hemochromatosis. What if you improve the condition of a thousand women and kill only one man, what if you help

20,000 women and still kill only one man, where is the break-even point in this trade-off?"

Another physician, Dr. Frederick Stohlman, Jr., chief of medicine and research at Boston's St. Elizabeth's Hospital and editor-in-chief of the professional magazine *Blood*, has fought the iron-enriching program bitterly, saying "This would be tantamount to an experiment on man on a national scale." Dr. Stohlman also mentions that victims of colon cancer frequently have a first symptom of iron deficiency anemia. Presumably their intestinal condition is such that they cannot absorb iron from their food. How will the doctor suspect cancer in these patients if they are getting so much iron in their food that they have no anemia? asks Dr. Stohlman.

Dr. Ogden Johnson, director of the FDA's Division of Nutrition, answers that he is aware of all these objections. "We've considered both sides for more than a year," he says. "A ten-state survey has shown that hemoglobin levels are often less and iron intake often less than believed consistent with optimal health. Many hemotologists see no danger here. We're setting a level less than recommended. Physicians can guide susceptible patients to special bread."

Finally, on October 13, 1973, the FDA announced that they had concluded more than three years of study by deciding that, if bakers want to label their bread "enriched," they must add additional iron—25 milligrams per pound of enriched bread—up from 8 to 12½ milligrams. But, as of now, the matter has still not been officially settled.

As we go to press there is still no certainty as to whether or not this great increase in iron enrichment of bread will go through.

During World War II the federal government insisted on "enriching" white bread with the three B vitamins that we have the most scientific information about— thiamine (B1), riboflavin (B2) and niacin (B3)—plus iron. Bakers did not have to comply with the federal enrichment program. But 30 states have made it mandatory that white bread sold in these states be "enriched." In all other states most bakers voluntarily add the vitamins and iron. However, other bakery products than bread are usually not enriched—rolls, pastries, etc.

U. S. Department of Agriculture Handbook No. 8, *Composition of Foods,* tells us that a serving of modern bread contains the following amounts of iron at present:

Cracked wheat	1.1 milligrams
French or Vienna (enriched)	2.2 "
Italian (enriched)	2.2 "
Raisin bread	1.3 "
Rye bread	1.6 "
Pumpernickel	2.4 "
White (enriched)	2.4 "
Whole wheat	2.3 "

This means, of course, that commercial whole wheat bread contains less iron than commercial, enriched white bread. One can only guess at the amount of actual wholegrain flour there must be in such "wholewheat" bread, for real wholewheat flour contains from 3.1 to 4.3 milligrams of iron. On the other hand, wheat bran contains 14.9 milligrams of iron and wheat germ contains 9.4 milligrams of iron.

Regardless of how much iron the bakers finally put in bread, it should not be of too much concern to the health seeker who is careful about what he eats. First of all, he should be baking his own bread at home. Second, he should eat plenty of meat, liver, eggs, whole-grain cereals, nuts and seeds, wheat germ and bran, green, leafy vegetables—all rich in iron. The true health seeker does not habitually buy commercial baker's bread or bakery products, whether or not they are enriched with additional iron. He either bakes his own or buys them at the health food store. So why bring up this matter at all?

We brought it up because we think it illustrates again and very effectively the terrible dilemma we get into as soon as we begin to tinker with food on a national basis. Taking all the iron out of cereal products and breads in the milling and baking causes widespread anemia, partly because of this deficiency. Then, too, our giant food industry has crammed the shelves of supermarkets, candy stores and drug stores with thousands of non-nourishing foods which, with astronomical advertising budgets, they persuade our people to eat. The result—nationwide malnutrition—in this case, iron-deficiency anemia. You simply can't cure it with a nationwide program of "enrichment." Those people whose inborn defect causes them to store too much iron will probably eat the enriched bread and get sicker. The people who really need the iron most will probably go right on living on soft drinks, potato chips, beer, pizza, cakes, candy, etc. The only way to cure nationwide iron deficiency is an education program which will guarantee that everyone knows, from childhood on, which foods to eat for good health and which to avoid.

The body may require 20 to 30 milligrams of iron daily. As we have discovered, much of this is iron which is saved by the body and used again. The rest of it must come from the diet or food supplements. Although there may be plenty of iron in a person's diet, it has been discovered that only about 10 per cent of the iron in food is absorbed. If you are certain you are getting enough iron in your food, can you be sure you will not have iron deficiency anemia? Not necessarily. People who suffer from disorders which interfere with their absorption of food may lack iron, no matter if their diets contain enough. Steatorrhea, chronic diarrhea, intestinal parasites, or worms, interfere with absorption of iron. And, as we mentioned, so do disorders which involve bleeding (ulcers, hemorrhoids, chronic nose bleeds.)

You must be certain, too, that your diet contains plenty of the other food elements which apparently help the body to use iron well: chiefly, vitamin C, copper, the B vitamins and protein. The iron of food is much better absorbed in an acid medium, which suggests that people who don't have enough of the acid digestive juices in their stomachs may suffer from lack of iron. A good, nourishing diet, especially rich in the B vitamins, will probably maintain the digestive juices adequately.

Earlier we mentioned the necessity of eating whole-grain breads and cereals, especially those sold in the health food store. As for those worthless cereals sold in the supermarket, here is what Dr. Jean Mayer said in a statement before the United States Senate Select Committee on Nutrition and Human Needs, March 5, 1973, in Washington, D. C.:

"The debasement of the food supply through advertising unfortunately is often true within groups. Let me make it clear that I think that some of the older-established cereals—hot cereals in particular, but many others as well—are excellent foods, the consumption of which should be encouraged for both children and adults. In particular, at a time when cardiovascular diseases are a major threat to the health of the nation, such cereals, consumed if need be with low fat milk, are an excellent breakfast replacement for high-cholesterol foods.

"Unfortunately, those cereals most heavily advertised to children are sugar-coated cereals (a number of which contain over 50 per cent sugar and, therefore, ought not to be properly called cereals.) According to the testimony of many young mothers, these are often eaten like candy, without milk. In spite of their being enriched with some vitamins and iron, the total effect is one of inadequate nutrition (deficient, in particular, in trace minerals—there are suggestions that zinc deficiency may be appearing among U. S. children, including middle and upper socioeconomic class children; chromium deficiency may be a factor among the elderly.)

"The promotion of high-fat, high-salt snacks to adults compounds cardiovascular risks," Dr. Mayer continues. "The promotion of high-sugar cereals, snacks and soft drinks to children is a dental disaster, and may be a factor in increasing the likelihood of diabetes in genetically vulnerable subjects; for the past two years consumption of sugar and corn syrup has exceeded our flour consumption—with unpredictable results for the health of the country."

How much iron do you need? The Recommended Daily Dietary Allowances, revised 1974, are:

Infants (to five months) .... 10 mg.
Infants (five months to 1 year) .... 15 mg.
Children (1 to 3 years) .... 15 mg.
Children (4 to 10 years) .... 10 mg.
Males (11 to 18 years) .... 18 mg.
Males (19 and over) .... 10 mg.
Females (11 to 50 years) .... 18 mg.
Females (51 and over) .... 10 mg.
Pregnant women .... 18 mg. and up
   (The National Research Council notes that this increased requirement cannot be met by ordinary diet; therefore, the use of supplemental iron is recommended.)
Lactating women .... 18 mg.

CHAPTER 10

Magnesium

"A 33-YEAR-OLD WOMAN sat in her doctor's office feeling very depressed," write Dr. John Prutting and Pat Curtis in the March 1971 issue of *Family Circle*. "Her physical complaints were that she felt tired and weak. But what upset her most was that she couldn't remember things the way she used to and felt unable to cope with her household. She had what is sometimes called 'housewife blues.'

"Her doctor listened to her complaints, examined her, went over her chart and questioned her about her diet," the article—"The Miracle Mineral That Keeps You Fit"—continues. "A blood test confirmed his suspicions. The woman was suffering from a deficiency of a very important mineral, magnesium.

"The doctor gave her magnesium by injection and put her on a high-magnesium diet. Within two weeks her symptoms had cleared. She felt more energetic, she could handle her housework and she could remember names and appointments as well as ever.

"This woman's condition—magnesium deficiency—is not unusual. But her doctor's recognition of it is the result of relatively new findings about this important mineral," the article says. Dr. Prutting adds that "Seventy per cent of us have mismanaged our diets enough to have some degree of magnesium deficiency." And Adelle Davis, writing in *Better Nutrition*, believes that "apparently everyone in America has a magnesium deficiency."

MAGNESIUM

In the July-August 1973 issue of the *National Health Federation Bulletin,* Dr. Michael Walczak of Studio City, Calif., says: "Magnesium activates more enzymes in the body than any other mineral. Among other things, it is also intimately involved in the storage of sugar as glycogen in the liver—and in its release into the blood for energy. Yet the so-called balanced diet' provides only about 25 per cent of the amount required for good health," Dr. Walczak says.

Dr. Gustave Standig-Lindberg, writing in *Medical World News,* October 13, 1972, believes that magnesium may be responsible for the brain damage that occurs in alcoholism. The Swedish researcher added that, even when DTs (delirium tremens) are present, brain tissues are not damaged, providing the alcoholic is getting enough magnesium. The damage can be reversed, in its early stages by "aggressive" magnesium therapy, Dr. Standig-Lindberg said.

The capillaries (the tiny blood vessels) are apt to be destroyed if there is too little magnesium in the body. When the capillaries in the nervous system are damaged, the brain, of course, is also affected.

Dr. Prutting tells us he has found that anyone who drinks heavily every day is probably deficient in magnesium. And he reminds us that the more high-protein foods you eat, the more magnesium you need. If you are taking large amounts of calcium, you tend to lose magnesium, for these two compete for absorption. Excess sugar in the diet can also cause you to lose magnesium. Dr. Prutting describes a patient who came to him many years ago complaining of repeated attacks of irregular heart beat—so devastating that they incapacitated him. His condition worsened when he drank anything alcoholic. Tests showed his blood level of magnesium to be very low. Injections and a diet high in magnesium cured all his symptoms. He is now able to drink moderately, but maintains always a high-magnesium diet.

Dairy Council Digest states that, in the past, experts believed that deficiency in magnesium was very rare among people who are fed as well as Americans, but "As food processing changes and the use of formulated foods increases, such assurance may not always be warranted." The *Digest* believes that we are eating less grain products than we used to, and this may be the reason why deficiency in this essential mineral is being uncovered more and more frequently.

Magnesium is needed for many processes that take place inside our bodies. It is intimately concerned with the way we use calcium, potassium and sodium. Magnesium is present in all living tissues. It is part of the chlorophyll molecule in plants. It is needed for the contraction of muscles. And remember that the heart is a muscle. It is needed for the sending of nerve impulses, which means that deficiency can produce nervous disorders, poor memory, irritability. Magnesium is required for the body to manufacture protein, fat and other essentials which make up cells and intercellular material.

It seems that magnesium may be useful in preventing unwanted calcification, like bladder and kidney stones. In animal experiments scientists have found that deficiency of magnesium will produce kidney stones. They have found that a chronically alkaline urine, and reduced excretion of magnesium will produce kidney stones. On diets low in magnesium, but high in phosphorus and moderate in calcium, calcification occurred in both heart and kidney. This kind of diet is rather common in our country, where the amount of phosphorus in meat dishes of all kinds tends to overbalance the amount of magnesium, which is found most abundantly in seed foods. So it seems that, when the diet is high in phosphorus, you need more magnesium for good balance.

"About 70 per cent of the magnesium in the body is in the bones," states *Food*, the Yearbook of Agriculture, 1959. "The rest is in the soft tissues and blood. Muscle tissue contains more magnesium than calcium. Blood contains more calcium than magnesium.

"Magnesium acts as starter or catalyzer for some of the chemical reactions within the body. It also becomes a part of some of the complex molecules that are formed as the body uses food for growth and for maintenance and repair. It plays an important role as a coenzyme in the building of protein. There is some relation between magnesium and the hormone cortisone as they affect the amount of phosphate in the blood."

We know that conditions of disease or stress cause us to need more magnesium, as we need more of many nutrients under such conditions. And there are some chronic ailments which cause us to lose magnesium, so anyone suffering from these should take special care to get

---

Magnesium in One Serving of Foods
100 grams or about ¼ pound

	Milligrams		Milligrams
Almonds	270	Molasses	
Apricots, raw	62	(blackstrap)	50
Asparagus, raw	20	Oats, wholegrain	169
Banana, raw	33	Peanuts	206
Barley, whole grain	124	Peanut butter	
Beans, lima	67	(⅓ cup)	82
Beets	25	Peanut flour	360
Beet greens	106	Peas	35
Brazilnuts	225	Pecans	142
Brussels sprouts	29	Pistachios	158
Cashew nuts	267	Rice, brown	88
Chard, Swiss	65	Rye flour	73
Corn, fresh	147	Sesame seeds	181
Cottonseed flour	650	Soybeans	265
Cowpeas		Soybean flour	
(blackeyed)	55	defatted	310
Dandelion greens	36	Walnuts	190
Filberts	184	Wheat bran	490
Lentils	80	Wheat germ	336
Millet	162	Whey, dried	130
		Yeast, brewer's	231

---

plenty of magnesium daily. These conditions are: any kidney disorders, diseases in which food is badly absorbed (diarrhea, colitis, etc.), hyperthyroidism, acute alcoholism, diabetes, disorders of the parathyroid gland. It is true, too, that anyone taking diuretics or any reason should be most conscious of the great loss of magnesium which this causes. Many people today are using diuretics in reducing pills. Many women use them to prevent accumulation of fluid preceding menstruation.

In her book, *Let's Get Well*, Adelle Davis relates magnesium to the following: hardening of the arteries, fatty substances in blood, epilepsy, chorea, alcoholism, diuretics, anemia, arthritis, bone abnormalities, celiac disease, diarrhea, excessive calcium intake, fatigue, insomnia, kidney disease, leg cramps, liver damage, loss of hair, muscle abnormalities, nervousness, personality changes, sensitivity to noise and pain, spastic constipation, tics, tremors, twitching, heart attacks, kidney stones.

Some nutrition experts are pressing for the addition of magnesium to white bread and flour, along with the several vitamins and iron which are now restored in the "enrichment" program. One reason is that lack of magnesium, as we have noted, is suspected as a contributing cause of heart disease and other circulatory problems.

Four Chicago investigators, writing in the March 27, 1967 issue of the *Journal of the American Medical Association*, described their experiments which seem to show that lack of magnesium may be involved as one of the causes of one kind of leukemia, or cancer of the blood. Working with a species of rat which is generally free from leukemia, the physicians kept the animals on a diet deficient in magnesium for eight or more months. Ten per cent of the rats developed leukemia, which was indistinguishable from that which victimizes human beings.

Over quite long periods of time diets were fed to different groups of rats, some including enough magnesium, others deficient in the mineral. At the same time, chemicals known to produce leukemia and/or cancer were fed to certain of the rats. The rats which got enough magnesium appeared to be immune to leukemia, although some of them succumbed to cancer. But those which did not get enough magnesium succumbed to leukemia and developed other ailments as well—trouble in the bone marrow, the kidneys, the heart and the muscles. By giving them plenty of magnesium, these latter symptoms could be cured. But not the leukemia. In addition, it appears that lack of magnesium may be responsible for mutations—that is, rats which lack the mineral may bear deficient children.

Says the *Journal*, "Conceivably, the research might lead to a search for a similar metabolic defect in humans." This is a curious word to use in relation to simple lack of magnesium in the diet. It seems to us that it was not a defect in the rats which caused them to get leukemia, but a defect in the diet!

We will undoubtedly have to wait for years before we hear any more about the possible relation of magnesium deficiency and leukemia. That's the way medical research works out. But, meanwhile, why not make sure you are getting enough magnesium, just in case some peculiarity in diet may have resulted in a shortage?

Studies of sick babies reported in *Lancet* for April 1, 1967 indicated that lack of appetite, delayed healing of wounds and tendency to feel cold all the time were typical. The author says that such conditions are possible "in view of the immense importance of the (magnesium) ion in energy production in almost every type of cell."

Two Japanese physicians, in the November 25, 1967 *Lancet*, reported on the possible relation of magnesium and thyroid disorders. A 1968 series of articles in the *New England Journal of Medicine* discussed this mineral in relation to parathyroid diseases, conditions of the adrenal glands, diabetes, bone cancers, pancreatitis, kid-

113

ney disorders and thyroid disorders. And a 1968 issue of *Endocrinology* reported on the theory of a Canadian physician that lack of magnesium may be related to cancer incidence. A high fat diet, he says, will cause much magnesium to be excreted and lots of us eat too much fat.

In *Medical Tribune*, October 3, 1968, a California physician relates lack of magnesium to ulcerations of skin, calcium deposits in muscles in both the skeleton and the heart, calcium deposits in kidneys, alterations in heart beat. A March 16, 1970 issue of *Medical Tribune* related lack of magnesium and zinc in the diet of pregnant animals to severe malformation or death of unborn offspring. A lack of these two minerals prevailing for only a short time can affect a high percentage of the unborn babies.

In a new book, *Vitamin B6: The Doctor's Report* (Harper & Row, New York), Dr. John M. Ellis and James Presley devote over seven pages to magnesium, especially as it relates to pyridoxine (B6). Dr. Ellis reports the case of a 62-year-old woman who complained of painful cramps and spasms of the arms and hands, feet and legs. In the clinic, he adds, muscle spasms in the legs, feet, arms and hands provide the best evidence of mineral imbalance. The four horsemen of metallic exchange at the cell level are magnesium, calcium, sodium and potassium, he says.

"The patient had many of the same symptoms of numbness and tingling that so often had proved responsive to pyridoxine," Dr. Ellis says. "Her fingers were painfully bowed at the metacarpophalangeal joints in both hands. Clinicians call this 'carpal spasms.' During flexion her finger joints popped and snapped, probably caused by the simultaneous pull of the tendons in extending and flexing the hands. She also had some terrible teeth; all of her lower incisors were decayed. Generally miserable for some time, she had suffered painful muscle spasms and had slept little over the past week. During the past two weeks she had been eating little but milk and soups.

"While still in my office," Dr. Ellis continues, "she was given two tablets that contained magnesium and potassium asparate. By the time she reached her home in a taxicab, her muscle spasms had subsided. The tablets contained a total of 500 milligrams of magnesium asparate and 500 milligrams of potassium asparate—about one half day's supply of each mineral, which she could have gotten from green vegetables if she had been able to eat them.

"She was given the magnesium and potassium tablets every six hours for 48 hours. She was relieved of spasms and pain. But her most valuable benefit may have been her improved sleep, for she was positive that her sound sleep thereafter was unusual and came as a result of the magnesium and potassium supplements.

"One practical application seems clear," Dr. Ellis concludes. "If a person cannot chew raw fruits and raw vegetables, he or she needs the juices of the raw vegetables. Dietitians, especially those who are employed in nursing homes where there are so many aged and debilitated persons, need to work diligently with delectable blends of juices from raw vegetables and fruits."

An article in the *Journal of the American Dietetic Association*, May 1970, analyzes the average hospital diet. The author found that many diets, especially salt-poor diets, low-calorie diets and low-protein and "soft" diets were woefully lacking in many important minerals. Magnesium was one of the minerals having "much lower values" than the amount specified officially as essential for good health. If dieticians in a hospital, with all the charts, scales, computers and mathematical formulas to guide them, cannot serve meals to very sick people which contain even the bare minimum of essential minerals, how much more likely is it that the average person will be short on minerals, since he has no knowledge of nutrition and no guide for choosing the right foods? If one is on a restrictive diet, one is much more likely to be short on essential minerals, without the most careful kind of planning of every meal.

"While no one knows why heart disease is so prevalent, it is highly probable that a primary cause lies in the fact that in our industrialized age the public chooses its food only on the basis of appearance and taste, and has not been educated to choose on the basis of nutritional value," states Dr. Roger J. Williams, the eminent nutrition expert at the University of Texas. His statement was part of a minority report that he sent to President Nixon's Advisory Panel on Heart Disease. He also pleaded for two or more National Institutes of Nutritional Science.

"The sins of omission occasioned by modern industrialization of food production without adequate regard for nutritional value are many. Among the essential nutrient items likely to be deficient or out of balance in the super-market produce commonly consumed are vitamin B6, magnesium, vitamin E, vitamin C, folic acid and trace minerals. This is not a complete list, but these items all appear to be involved in the heart disease problem. All these and other nutrient items are needed to keep the cells and tissues of hearts and blood vessels healthy," Dr. Williams says.

Since the four essential minerals—calcium, sodium, potassium and magnesium—are so intricately intertwined and interbalanced in their functions in the human body, there is danger of creating imbalances if you get too much or too little of any one. The solution, of course, is to eat as widely varied a diet as possible, and to depend on natural foods for the minerals, since, in wholly natural foods, this important balance has not been disturbed.

When flour is refined, for example, most of the magnesium is removed, when the bran and germ are removed. White bread contains 22 milligrams of magnesium, compared to commercial whole wheat which contains 78 milligrams. And, of course, commercial whole wheat bread depends on white flour for a large part of its ingredients. So real whole-grain bread is bound to have a lot more magnesium, since the entire wheat berry is in the flour of which it is made.

The best sources of magnesium are seeds of all kinds, and this, of course, includes nuts and whole grains. Says the previously mentioned *Family Circle* article, "Wheat germ, wheat bran, oatmeal, corn and cornmeal are excellent. Mothers of young children should be glad to hear that peanut butter is high on the list of magnesium-rich foods." Brewers yeast runs a close second to wheat bran in its magnesium content, and soybeans—those delicious legumes on which vegetarians depend for much of their protein—have almost as much magnesium as wheat germ.

In planning diets to assure yourself of enough magnesium, it is well to take into account the amount of the various foods one customarily eats at a meal. A fourth of a pound of peanuts contains about the same amount of magnesium as a fourth of a pound of peanut butter. You can eat a fourth of a pound of peanuts without much trouble. That much peanut butter might be too much to handle. So it's wise to use the peanut butter—and almond and other nut butters—in preparing many other foods. They add flavor and nutriment to soups, salads, casseroles, baked goods, desserts, etc. Blackstrap molasses, almost as rich in magnesium as wheat bran, is not consumed by the quarter pound. But you can use small amounts of it to enrich many foods—milk drinks, puddings, whole-grain goods, etc. Remember, it has a stronger molasses taste than other molasses.

The chart shows you the amount of magnesium in many common foods. Note how many of these are seed foods, and include plenty of them at every meal as well as in-between-meal snacks.

The 1974 Recommended Daily Dietary Allowances for

magnesium—which are issued by the Food and Nutrition Board of the National Academy of Sciences-National Research Council in Washington, D.C.—are:

Infants	60 to 70 mg.
Children (1 to 3)	150 mg.
Children (4 to 6)	200 mg.
Children (7 to 10)	250 mg.
Males (11 to 14)	350 mg.
Males (15 to 18)	400 mg.
Males (19 and over)	350 mg.
Females (all ages)	300 mg.
Pregnant and lactating females	450 mg.

CHAPTER 11

Zinc

WHEN WE THINK of zinc—which is a bluish-white substance resembling magnesium—we are apt to think in terms of galvanized sheets, battery cells, roof coverings and a variety of industrial applications. But the trace mineral zinc is an important cog in the complex human nutritional machinery. And many competent nutritionists, such as Dr. Jean Mayer of Harvard University, believe that many people in the United States have a zinc deficiency.

In testimony before the U.S. Senate Select Committee on Nutrition and Human Needs, April 30, 1973, in Washington, D.C., the following exchange was made between Senator Richard Schweiker (R., Pa.), a member of the committee, and Dr. Walter Mertz, Chairman, Human Nutrition Institute, U.S. Department of Agriculture:

DR. MERTZ. It is my experience, and I have no logical explanation for it, that whenever a population becomes more well-to-do that there is a trend toward more fancy foods, there is a trend for eating increasing proportion of the meals outside the house. Now, a poor population is more or less forced to live with very little processing. We have not yet learned to understand the optimum requirement for all essential trace nutrients. Therefore, if we fabricate our own foods, we must accept that our knowledge is incomplete and, therefore, it is entirely possible that our fabricated foods are inferior in quality to that of the more wholesome products.

SENATOR SCHWEIKER. In your statement, Doctor, you refer to the National Nutritional Survey which finds there is widespread iron deficiency anemia in the country. I know in an affluent society a finding like this comes as a great shock to many people. Since we have had iron fortification policy in this country for many years, why, in your judgment, was the fortification policy inadequate, and what shall we do to correct it?

DR. MERTZ. The fortification policy was less than a full success because when we instituted it, we did not have enough basic knowledge about the availability of different iron compounds. At that time we thought that any iron salt is equal to any other iron salt. In the meantime we have learned that there are certain iron compounds which are very poorly available and others much better available. We have not incorporated this knowledge into our enrichment program of years ago. Here, again, in the past 5 to 10 years, basic nutrition has produced knowledge of certain iron compounds that are available to man and that can be incorporated into foods and that will hopefully improve the enrichment program.

SENATOR SCHWEIKER. You refer to the fact, in your statement, that people need less calories and eat less in an industrialized society. Also, that in such a situation they are more likely to end up deficient in various micronutrients. Can you give us another example besides iron?

DR. MERTZ. Yes. I would say that we certainly have an example in zinc nutrition. In the past 5 to 10 years there has accumulated evidence that the zinc nutrition status of a proportion of our older population is not optimal as shown by very good effects of increasing zinc intake. For example, in hospitalized patients. We are now seeing new evidence that ties the zinc nutritional status to the impairment of taste acuity, which is an extremely important factor, particularly in children. Last year evidence was produced indicating that approximately 8 to 10 per cent of a number of supposedly normal children from middle—or high-income neighborhoods examined were markedly zinc deficient, as evidenced by poor taste acuity, poor appetite and so forth. (End of quote).

About 100 years ago a researcher named J. Raulin showed that zinc is essential for the life of a small organism. Not until 1926 did we know that higher forms of life need it also. Eventually we learned that zinc is necessary for a wide range of processes in living cells. An average 150-lb. man has in his body only about 1 or 2 grams of zinc, which is about half the amount of iron his body contains; 15 times more than his copper supply; 100 times more than the manganese his body contains.

Nutrition experts used to believe that it was impossible for human beings to develop deficiency in zinc, since it is so widespread in food and water. But now we know differently, says an editorial in the *Lancet* for February 10, 1973. Zinc deficiency has been found in badly nourished people; it disappears rapidly from the body under certain kinds of stress, and zinc can also be used for various healing purposes.

Zinc is needed for bone growth. Lack of zinc in national diets has produced a dwarfed condition along with failure of sex organs to develop. When these individuals were given zinc supplements, they began to grow and sex organs matured. The deficiency of zinc was caused not so much by lack of the mineral in food as by the fact that the diet consisted almost entirely of cereal in which phytic acid was abundant. This element causes the minerals in food to be incompletely absorbed.

Studying zinc amounts in hospital food, several researchers found that "good quality" hospital diets gave an average of about 7 to 16 milligrams of zinc daily. Foods rich in protein were better sources of the mineral than refined carbohydrate foods. Because such a large part of modern diet consists of refined carbohydrate foods, there is a great possibility that many modern diets are deficient in zinc.

Zinc seems to help in healing certain kinds of wounds. Some researchers theorize this may be because the hospitalized patients were short on zinc to begin with, so all the zinc supplements are doing is to restore the normal values. How much zinc to give to correct a deficiency or to spur wound healing is not known. But there seems to be no indication that zinc is ever harmful.

One reason why giving zinc may be helpful in getting wounds to heal is that wounds, bone fractures and operations cause the body to lose large amounts of zinc in urine. Gordon S. Fell of the Royal Infirmary, Glasgow, Scotland, says that any disease or condition of starvation which causes a loss of muscle (untreated diabetes, for example) also causes zinc to be excreted. Skeletal muscle contains about 63 per cent of all body zinc. The total losses are large, Dr. Fell told the Ninth International Congress of Nutrition in October 1972, and could lead to zinc deficiency in severe cases. Other nutrients as well are excreted under such conditions: nickel, potassium, nitrogen and magnesium.

It is possible to raise the zinc levels in various organs and parts of the body by taking zinc supplements. If one wants to theorize on which parts of the body seem most dependent on a goodly supply of zinc, it is wise to take a look at where the trace mineral is concentrated. For example, the male prostate gland contains more zinc than any other organ of the human body—102 micrograms per gram—almost twice as much as the liver and kidney. All body muscles—including the heart—store zinc, indicating that this mineral is apparently very important to the healthful operation of muscles and heart. The pancreas, lung, spleen, brain, testes and adrenal glands also contain appreciable amounts of zinc.

Dr. E. J. Underwood, in *Trace Elements in Human and Animal Nutrition,* says that the zinc content of the pancreas is especially interesting since this mineral seems to play a part in the manufacture of insulin, which is the hormone that helps to control blood sugar levels. The vascular coating of the eye contains more zinc than any other part of the body, says Dr. Underwood, and other parts of the eye also contain this mineral. Scientists do not know what role the mineral plays in eye health.

The male sex organs of mammals are extraordinarily high in zinc, notably the prostate gland, which is where the male sperm is stored. The sperm cells are also high in zinc.

The addition of zinc to insulin solutions given to diabetics delays the action of insulin, so that the diabetic has a longer period of lowered blood sugar, hence does not need more insulin quite so soon.

Zinc supplements have been given to people suffering from hardening of the arteries. In one study, some of the patients showed considerable improvement. Others were so greatly improved that they could return to their usual activities.

Researchers at the University of Cincinnati Medical Center believe that the answer to high blood levels of cholesterol may be to raise levels of zinc and copper. Dr. Harold G. Petering and his colleagues (Dr. Lalitha Murthy and Dr. Ellen J. O'Flaherty) found that, when zinc and copper levels of blood rise, fat levels decrease. Dr. Petering says, "These findings might help to unravel some of the problems of environmental health. If man is subjected to certain environmental conditions, such as exposure to a chemical that depresses zinc and copper, he might also get elevated levels of lipids (fats)." He thinks that the human being may be especially susceptible to damage from cholesterol because "he may have enough zinc and copper in his body to get good growth but not enough to forestall high and potentially dangerous levels of blood fats." Dr. Petering's research was reported in a press release from the National Institutes of Health,

October 25, 1972. One environmental metal which is a zinc antagonist is cadmium which, as we will find out in a later chapter, is prevalent in air pollution in most cities —and especially abundant in the lead and cadmium pollution in heavy traffic.

A relationship between zinc in adrenal glands and the amount of cholesterol in those glands was discovered by a Scots researcher and reported in *Proceedings of the Nutrition Society*, September 1972. Laboratory rats kept on diets deficient in zinc had more cholesterol in their adrenal glands than those kept on diets containing plenty of this mineral. The adrenal glands are two ductless glands located above the kidneys; they secrete at least two hormones—adrenalin and cortin.

Absence of the sense of taste, as noted earlier by Dr. Walter Mertz, was found in some children who had low levels of zinc. This was discovered during a survey of how much zinc they had in their hair. Measuring trace minerals in hair is an acceptable way of determining the body store. Ten children out of 338 apparently normal children were found to have low amounts of zinc in their hair. Five of these had almost no sense of taste. (Doctors call this hypogeusia.) They also had poor appetites. They were given zinc supplements and, after three months, appetites returned to normal and sense of taste returned as well. Four scientists report these experiments in *Pediatric Research*, Vol. 6, page 868, 1972.

In 1968, Dr. William B. Bean of the Department of Internal Medicine at the University of Iowa said that there is some evidence that diets deficient in zinc may set the stage for rheumatoid arthritis. Chicks fed diets deficient in zinc developed bone enlargements and deformities that resemble human arthritis. And deficiency in zinc causes an increase in congenital deformities in animals.

A Greek scientist (Research Laboratory of Physiopathology of Animal Reproduction, Athens) reported in a letter to the editor of *Lancet,* December 9, 1972 that he had noticed in himself an unexplained result of taking zinc supplements.

Says Dr. F. N. Demertzis, "Working recently with zinc, I was impressed with the effect of zinc supplements on apparently healthy animals. So I decided to take zinc myself. The result was surprising. Firstly the long hairs of the eyebrows (a sign of the aged) disappeared, and new, short and thin adolescent-like eyebrows took their place. The hair became more healthy and shining, its color darker, and every trace of dandruff disappeared. In the comb in the morning there was not a single hair anymore. Finally the greasy skin (full of acne at the time of my adolescence) became dry and better than I had ever had it. After my experience, the same effect was noted in three other people I know who took zinc."

Women who take The Pill should increase their vitamin intake or risk becoming anemic, according to Dr. Rosalind Alfin-Slater, Professor of Nutrition and Biochemistry at the University of California at Los Angeles. Dr. Alfin-Slater said that the nutrients which are especially important are vitamin B2 (riboflavin), folic acid, vitamin E and certain minerals such as zinc and chromium. She said, too, that women on the oral contraceptive may not just become anemic if they are short on nutrients. They can also develop certain skin ailments. Her remarks before the American Oil Chemists Society meeting were reported in the June 17, 1973 issue of *Parade.*

A University of Rochester scientist has revealed that zinc is essential not only for proper healing of wounds, but also for the treatment of arteriosclerosis (hardening of the arteries). In 36 patients treated with doses of zinc, 30 showed improvement in being able to exercise longer and an increased warmth of feet and hands. Fourteen developed pulses where none had existed before.

"These results are very encouraging," says Dr. Walter

J. Pories, "because atherosclerosis is a disease which generally becomes progressively worse and rarely shows spontaneous improvement." In addition to artery disease, low zinc levels may also be associated with cirrhosis and lung cancer.

Nature, the most prestigious science journal in the world, which is published in London, reported in its June 18, 1971 issue that laboratory animals given a supplement containing 22 parts per million of zinc were able to withstand a cancer-causing drug which caused tumors in a second group of animals which did not get the zinc supplement. The article concludes that giving zinc as a dietary supplement "seems to exert an inhibitory effect on tumor formation."

It is no longer news that many doctors and psychiatrists are successfully treating schizophrenia, our most serious mental disorder, with megadoses of B vitamins and vitamin C. Now a New Jersey psychiatrist has reported that supplements of zinc and manganese also appear to have a beneficial effect. As reported in *Medical Tribune*, Dr. Carl C. Pfeiffer of the New Jersey Neuropsychiatric Institute, Stillman, N.J., told an international Symposium on Clinical Applications of Zinc Metabolism that "a probable factor in some of the schizophrenias is a combined deficiency of zinc and manganese, with a relative increase in iron or copper or both."

Copper is excreted very poorly by many victims of this terrible disease, he said. And often high levels of copper are associated with the disease. Copper is a zinc antagonist—that is, the more copper you have, the less zinc you are likely to have. About one-fifth of all the patients he examined had more copper in their blood than they should have and less zinc. Some patients had too much iron in their blood; some had too little. When the blood levels of copper increased, the disease grew worse. But when Dr. Pfeiffer gave his patients zinc and manganese supplements, copper was excreted and the proper balance between the two minerals was obtained.

Dr. Pfeiffer was especially enthusiastic about using the zinc-manganese supplement with women and girls suffering from schizophrenia. Estrogen, the female sex hormone, is also associated with high levels of copper in the blood. In the mentally ill, these high levels of estrogen may actually approximate those of the ninth month of pregnancy, which are abnormally high. By giving the zinc-manganese supplement, the amounts of copper can be controlled.

The supplement is also valuable in some cases of mental depression because "this may herald the onset of schizophrenia." Though Dr. Pfeiffer does not mention it, zinc, as we know, is closely associated with high and low blood sugar levels in the diabetic state. And low blood sugar is one of the symptoms often found in schizophrenics. Vitamin C is destroyed by exposure to copper, either in the body or in a kitchen utensil. This may be one reason why massive doses of vitamin C have been found valuable for the mentally ill. Although the increased levels of copper in the blood may destroy some of it, enough is left to do all the important work which vitamin C must do in the body.

Two recent reports indicate the close relationship between zinc and two vitamins. *The Proceedings of the Nutrition Society* (May, 1973) tell us that, in animals, when there are low supplies of zinc, there may also be low liver concentrations of folic acid, the important but rather scarce B vitamin. And in *Science,* September 7, 1973, we discover that the amount of vitamin A available for use in the blood depends partly on the zinc status of the body. Zinc is essential, it seems, to "mobilize" vitamin A from the liver, so that it can perform its usual bodily functions. If there is not enough vitamin A in the blood to guarantee such activity, zinc supplements may call the vitamin out of the liver, as it were, and make it available to the rest of the body. As you see, the more we learn about trace minerals, the more complex their relationships become.

Writing in the September 7, 1973 issue of *Medical World News*, a Montreal, Canada group of researchers disclosed at a meeting of the American Neurological Association and the Canadian Congress of Neurological Sciences that one of the amino acids, taurine—a non-essential one—and zinc appear to be related to one's susceptibility to epileptic seizures. They do not, as yet, have definite information as to just how these two substances may function, but they are proceeding with further work along these lines. Amino acids are the building blocks of protein—the basic stuff of which we are made. Most of our interest centers on those which we call "essential," meaning that we must get them in food, since our bodies cannot manufacture them. But taurine is a non-essential amino acid—that is, the normal body can make it so there is no need to get it in food.

So how could anyone be deficient in taurine, if, indeed, we can make it ourselves without the necessity of getting it in food? One presumes that something in the epileptic's physiological make-up may prevent him from making his own taurine. In that case, giving the amino acid might repair the damage. Of course, it would have to be given for the rest of his life.

Working on this hypothesis, Dr. John Donaldson and Dr. André Barbeau of Montreal's Clinical Research Institute gave taurine to 12 epileptic patients who were having at least three seizures a day, although they were all taking maximum doses of conventional medicines. The seizures decreased in frequency within 24 hours and later were eliminated entirely, although the patients are still getting their anticonvulsant drugs. The doctors are not sure what level of the amino acid should be given, so they cannot suggest dosages for others.

The reasons why zinc may be important for this purpose are too complex for the layman to understand.

Basically, they have to do with the possibility that zinc may be involved in binding a certain substance in a certain part of the brain so that it is there to perform its function. It is well known that the amount of zinc in that part of the brain is considerable.

Looking further, the two doctors discovered that 32 of their epileptic patients had 15 per cent less zinc in their blood than non-epileptics. It seems to them that this trace mineral may work along with the amino acid to provide what is lacking in the make-up of the epileptic. Both doctors emphasize that their findings are very preliminary and they can give no definite answers as yet. But it looks hopeful.

As we have stated, prostate troubles are almost universal among older men in our part of the world and are becoming increasingly common among younger men as well. The gland swells and cuts off the flow of urine from the bladder, a condition so painful and so serious that an operation may be necessary. Prostate cancer is also a disease that is increasing. Isn't it possible that lack of this trace mineral zinc, which is apparently extremely important for the health of the prostate gland, may be at least part of the cause of this modern epidemic? Is it possible that the swelling of the prostate gland is reacting the same way the thyroid gland does when it desperately needs iodine?

For some reason, not yet understood, the levels of zinc in blood vary from one geographical region of the United States to another. Could this be because soil or drinking water in some parts of the country lack zinc? No final explanation has been made, but, in view of the fact that the amount of zinc available for human beings is "marginal," perhaps we should become concerned about this discrepancy.

In any event, most American men are brought up on diets in which processed cereals, white bread and other foods made of white flour are staples. Since the zinc has been removed from all these and never replaced, could not this single factor explain why prostate gland problems are so prevalent in Western society and almost unknown among more "backward" people who are still eating unprocessed, unrefined cereal products?

Writing on zinc in his syndicated column, Dr. Jean Mayer tells us that, in the light of zinc deficiencies that have been uncovered, "we are going to have to take another serious look at our diets and particularly at our methods of milling and enriching grain products. For zinc, like iron, is present in whole wheat. And, like iron, zinc is mostly eliminated. But, unlike iron, it is not being replaced by enrichment.

"If you want to play it safe," Dr. Mayer continues, ". . . there are many good sources of zinc. Foremost are fish and shellfish which have 10 to 100 times as much zinc as other foods. Moreover these foods are very good for you in other ways. Herring, oysters and clams are good sources. Quite a bit lower than fish, but still high in zinc, are cereals that are barely processed, such as oatmeal. Then there's liver, beef, whole wheat bread, peas, corn, egg yolk, dry yeast (brewers yeast), carrots, milk and rice."

We should make a regular daily practice of eating those foods in which all the trace elements are known to be abundant. Since trace elements are removed almost totally when sugarcane is refined and made into white sugar, and when grains are refined into processed cereals and white flour, we should omit these two categories of food at all our meals, and concentrate instead on the health-giving, well-balanced nourishment of the four main groups of food: meat, eggs, fish, poultry; dairy products of all kinds; fresh fruits and vegetables (chiefly those that are bright green and bright yellow), plus wholegrain cereals and breads and all nut and seed foods.

Although zinc has long been officially recognized as an essential nutrient for man, it was not until the new 1974

Recommended Daily Dietary Allowances were issued that we knew how much of this trace mineral we should be getting. The recommendations from the National Academy of Sciences are:

Infants (to five months) .... 3 mg.
Infants (Five months to 1 year) .... 5 mg.
Children (1 to 10) .... 10 mg.
Males and Females (all ages) .... 15 mg.
Pregnant Females .... 20 mg.
Lactating Females .... 25 mg.

CHAPTER 12

Sodium, Potassium, Chloride and Chlorine

In previous chapters we have discussed iron deficiency, zinc deficiency, calcium deficiency, magnesium deficiency, etc. In the United States, except under very unusual circumstances, it is unlikely that any of us will ever suffer a sodium or potassium deficiency. Although sodium and potassium are essential in human nutrition, dietary allowances have not been established because these two substances are readily available in the foods that we eat. Sodium occurs in many foods and sodium chloride (table salt) is often added to food to improve palatability or for preservation. As for potassium, typical diets will contain from 0.8 to 1.5 grams of potassium per 1,000 calories. An intake of this amount has been estimated to be near the minimal potassium need.

"Sodium, potassium and magnesium are essential in nutrition," states *Food*, The Yearbook of Agriculture, 1959. "They are among the most plentiful minerals in the body. Calcium and phosphorus are present in the largest amounts, and then come potassium, sulfur, sodium, chlorine and magnesium in descending order of amounts. A person who weighs 154 pounds has about 9 ounces of potassium, 4 ounces of sodium and 1.3 ounces of magnesium in his body."

Sodium is a soft, white, alkaline metallic chemical element which has a wax-like consistency. It is a constituent of many common compounds—sodium chloride (salt), sodium bicarbonate (baking powder), etc. Potassium is a silvery-white metallic substance.

"Sodium and potassium are similar in chemical properties but different in their location in the body," reports *Food*. "Sodium is chiefly in the fluids that circulate outside the cells, and only a small amount of it is inside the cells. Potassium is mostly inside the cells, and a much smaller amount in the body fluids. The interrelation between amounts of these minerals in their different locations permits substances to pass back and forth between the cells and the surrounding fluids. This process of exchange is called osmosis.

"Sodium and potassium are vital in keeping a normal balance of water between the cells and the fluids," *Food* continues. "Sodium and potassium are essential for nerves to respond to stimulation, for the nerve impulses to travel to the muscles, and for the muscles to contract. All types of muscles—including the heart—are influenced by sodium and potassium. These two elements also work with proteins, phosphates and carbonates to keep a proper balance between the amount of acid and alkali in the blood."

According to Adelle Davis, writing in *Let's Eat Right to Keep Fit*, potassium, sodium and chlorine are essential parts of the glandular secretions. We have noted the functions of sodium and potassium. Chlorine, she says, is used in forming hydrochloric acid in the stomach. These three nutrients are excreted daily in the urine, the amount being equal to that ingested by a healthy person, she adds. As we know, chlorine is used to treat water—it's a powerful bleaching agent—and, of course, it is an element in table salt (sodium chloride).

"Sodium and chlorine are amply supplied by table

salt," Miss Davis says. "Potassium is widely spread. . . . It is not enough, however, for sodium, chlorine and potassium to be adequate at all times; sodium and potassium must be in balance, each with the other. An excess of sodium causes much-needed potassium to be lost in the urine. The reverse is equally true: an excess of potassium can cause a serious loss of sodium. For example, herbivorous animals have such a high intake of potassium that they can retain little sodium; they die unless they can get salt. In early America, such animals were known to have walked hundreds of miles to salt licks. . . ."

She continues: "Under normal conditions, a healthy person runs little risk of deficiencies of sodium and chlorine. In extremely hot weather, however, so much salt can be lost through perspiration that death may result. Death from salt deficiency occurred during the first years of work on Boulder Dam and similar projects. During the blistering summer of 1933, I corresponded with an engineer who was working on Parker Dam. Each letter contained some such note as, 'We had a wonderful cook but he died yesterday of heatstroke.' The symptoms of sunstroke also are now recognized as caused largely by loss of salt through perspiration."

Salt depletion—"miner's cramps"—in industrial works was recorded in 1923, reports *Recommended Dietary Allowances*, 6th Revised Edition, 1964. The basis of this deficiency, characterized by nausea, vomiting, vertigo, mental apathy, exhaustion, cramps and respiratory failure, is failure to replace the salt losses during excessive sweating while the water losses are replaced.

"Workers in hot environments should have free access to water," states *Recommended Dietary Allowances*. "If more than 4 liters (a liter is 1.0567 U.S. liquid quarts) of water is consumed, extra salt should be provided, approximately 1 gram per liter of water. In addition to the losses in sweat, significant sodium depletion may be caused by vomiting or diarrhea or by urinary losses in

Foods with High Salt Content

Bacon
Beef, corned
Beef, dried
Bouillon cubes
Breads,
   commercial
Catsup
Caviar
Cheese
Codfish, salted
Cereals,
   commercial

Crackers,
   commercial
Ham
Herring,
   smoked
Hot dogs
Luncheon
   meats
Mustard
Olives
Pickles

Pizza
Popcorn,
   salted
Potato chips
Salad
   dressings,
   commercial
Salt pork
Salted nuts
Sausage
Soups, canned

patients with chronic renal (kidney) disease, or following the prolonged use of diuretics. Salt depletion also occurs in adrenocortical failure."

From the august pages of the *Journal of the American Medical Association,* April 29, 1968, comes a startling theory on the harmfulness of the large amounts of salt most of us modern Americans eat daily. The theory has its basis in evolution and patterns of eating that evolved with man as he evolved. An editorial in the *JAMA* discusses the theory of Prof. O. M. Helmer, who believes that too much salt does us harm for very good reasons closely related to our background and those ancient ancestors of ours who were vegetarians. Dr. Helmer theorizes that human beings must have been largely vegetarian, way back in history, because they had no weapons with which to kill animals for food.

A vegetarian diet contains large amounts of potassium and not much sodium. So, through all the many years that human beings were living largely on fruits, nuts and berries, their bodies learned that potassium was always plentiful, hence could be wasted. To this day, the body excretes a given amount of potassium in urine and perspiration daily. Even though the potassium content of one's diet may go down to almost nothing, tne body still goes right on excreting it, as if there were always plenty of it available. On the other hand, sodium is carefully "saved" by the body. If you restrict anyone's intake of sodium to much less than 500 milligrams daily, excretion of this mineral will stop almost completely because, theorizes Dr. Helmer, down through countless ages, mankind had so little sodium available that his body had to conserve it. Over many generations, only those humans survived who could carefully conserve enough sodium for good health. The rest perished. And the ability to conserve sodium was passed along to the next generation, and the next.

Then human beings discovered how to make weapons, and mankind became largely a hunter. The people who stayed in the tropical countries could get plenty of potassium from the fresh things that are available the year around. But, while they had enough sodium, the meat-eating human beings tended to lack potassium.

Today, thousands of generations away from those early men, most of us have comparatively enormous amounts of sodium in our diets—meat, eggs, dairy products and fish are all rich in this mineral and rather poor in potassium. And we salt everything we eat. Since our bodies learned over the ages to conserve sodium, we run into many problems associated with it. We simply do not excrete as much sodium as we should. And we eat far, far more than we need. Many physicians blame our widespread incidence of high blood pressure on the amount of salt we eat which is not excreted.

On the other hand, we are eating less and less of the foods that contain lots of potassium—fruits and vegetables and whole-grain cereal products. But our bodies are reckless in disposing of potassium.

In a letter to the editor of *Nutrition Reviews*, April 1968, Dr. Lewis K. Dahl of the Brookhaven National Laboratory remonstrates firmly with an earlier writer who challenged his contention that we are making salt addicts out of our children. Dr. Dahl says that human breast milk, on which human infants have been nourished since time immemorial, contains very little sodium. Cow's milk, on the other hand, contains about four or five times more sodium than human milk. So the baby who gets a bottle instead of being nursed begins life with four or five times more sodium than he needs. Then his mother is apt to feed him canned baby foods, which are heavily salted. There is obviously no need for these to be salted. The baby does not need any added salt on his food. In prepared baby foods, he gets vegetables and fruits with their high potassium content and he gets meat and eggs with their plentiful sodium content. So there is no physiological reason for him to get additional salt.

Salt was first added to baby food in 1931, reports *Be a Healthy Mother, Have a Healthy Baby*. "The salt added to practically all baby foods is put there more to appeal to the mother's taste than the baby's. He'll like it as well without salt." The book goes on to discuss Dr. Dahl's work at Brookhaven National Laboratory, Upton, N. Y., and states: "It's been established by L. K. Dahl and associates, on the basis of experiments with animals at Brookhaven, that too much salt in an infant's diet can lead to high blood pressure later in life. Young rats in Dahl's study, reported in *Review of Allergy* (September, 1970), developed permanent, even fatal, hypertension after brief exposures to excessive dietary salt found in commercial baby foods."

Dr. Dahl has carefully measured the amount of salt in prepared baby foods and has found that a day's ration of canned baby foods, plus the average amount of milk, gives the average baby an amount of sodium equivalent to 23 grams a day for an adult—almost twice the amount eaten by the average adult!

In *Nature* (October 6, 1962), three Johns Hopkins University scientists reported on tests of high blood pressure patients. They found that they cannot taste salt as well as those with normal blood pressure. The scientists believe, they said, that this may be one reason why hypertensive people often eat much larger amounts of salt than the rest of us.

A French physician is quoted in *Medical World News*, December 3, 1965, as saying that high blood pressure is more common among infants and children than anyone knows. He found hypertension in 24 children between the ages of 8 months to 18 years. In a number of cases the hypertension had already produced disorders of the kidneys. Placing the children on low-salt diets and giving them drugs brought the high blood pressure back to normal.

Writing to the editor of *Lancet*, January 9, 1965, a physician stated that many modern foods and drinks contain sodium of which we are not even aware: the sodium benzoate preservative used in many foods, sodium nitrate used in almost all meat products, and sodium added to butter, bread, cake, etc.

A Japanese scientist reported in *Geriatrics*, October, 1964, that strokes are the leading cause of death in Japan. Hypertension is more common there than in the United States. And the intake of salt, especially in one section of Japan, is considerably higher than it is here.

Another Japanese researcher, Yamaguchi, writing in the *Kobe Journal of Medical Sciences*, tells of laboratory experiments in which he induced high blood pressure in rats by giving them table salt for about 25 weeks. In another experiment, he gave the rats latent hypertension by certain laboratory procedures. Then he fed some of them a diet high in salt, while others were fed a diet low in salt. Those which got the most salt developed high blood pressure. Those which ate very little salt did not.

Dr. Garfield Duncan, an expert on the treatment of obesity, said in *Science News Letter*, June 29, 1963, that potato chips and pretzels, along with a dinner of salty ham, can raise your weight two or three pounds in one day. He also said that some of his patients who weighed as much as 300 pounds have lost as much as 10 pounds in one day simply by omitting salt. Since 15 to 20 per cent of his overweight patients have high blood pressure, there seems to be plenty of reason for incriminating salt as one reason for the high blood pressure as well as the obesity.

"A study to determine the salt intake habits of people with hypertension showed that those with high blood pressure consumed four times as much salt as a control group with normal pressure," reports *The New York Times*, September 11, 1973. "The 10 hypertensive and 12 normal patients were hospitalized for a week and fed dry diets with a choice of fluids—distilled water or equal amounts of salt water. The hypertensive group consumed four times the amount of salt as the normal group. They also took in twice the amount of fluid as the control group," the *Times* says. This study was conducted by Dr. Paul J. Schechter, Dr. David Horowitz and Dr. Robert I. Henkin, all of the National Heart and Lung Institute, and reported in the *Journal of the American Medical Association*.

A considerable number of Americans are on diets which restrict their intake of salt. Doctors usually restrict the salt in your diet if you are suffering from high blood pressure, congestive heart failure, kidney diseases, cardiopulmonary diseases (those involving heart and lungs), allergic states and liver disorders. According to an article in the *Archives of Environmental Health*, restriction of salt is an important part of therapy "during a large percentage of pregnancies."

For those people who must restrict salt in their diets, many diet foods are available at your health food store. There is here a large collection of common prepared foods to which salt has not been added during the preparation. There are nuts, seeds, bread, etc. Then, too, there are many different kinds of seasonings which are low in salt. Regardless of where you are shopping, always read labels to find out exactly what is in the product you are buying.

Since we eat salt only because we like its taste, it is fairly easy to shop in your health food store and find another seasoning whose taste pleases you as much as the taste of salt. There are mineral salt substitutes and there are many herbal mixtures which give a pleasant flavor to food without adding salt. Actually, salt, in the amounts in which many people eat it, can almost be said to be a drug, because its use actually has no relation to nutrition or need.

But suppose you have cut out as much salt as you can from your diet and have gone to a great deal of trouble to provide yourself with salt substitutes. What about the possibility of salt in your drinking water? The *Journal of the American Dietetic Association* published two articles on this subject which revealed some astonishing facts. The authors—all from the Public Health Service—tested the drinking water in 2,100 municipalities for two years. They found that the sodium in the water varied greatly from place to place. Most of the water supplies with very high sodium content are in the Far West and Midwest, they tell us, but they add that they found drinking waters of high sodium content in all areas of the United States.

They came to the conclusion that about 40 per cent of all municipal water supplies are not satisfactory to use, if your doctor has put you on a diet which restricts your daily intake of sodium to 500 milligrams. The drinking water which you use for cooking, too, would add so much sodium to your meals that the whole purpose of the diet would be negated.

The Archives of Environmental Health article which we referred to above, by Dr. Glen E. Garrison and Dr. O. L. Ader, shows the effect of water softeners on the salt content of drinking water. These men analyzed the drinking water of one community with a number of wells and found that the minimum amount of sodium in one well was 1 milligram per liter and the sodium content went all the way up to 137 milligrams per liter, with every possible variation in between. In a test of homes with water softeners, they found a thousand-fold difference in the amount of sodium in the water. Forty-eight of these homes had water which normally contained from 0 to 99 milligrams of sodium per liter. But after the water passed through a water softener, one of these homes had water which contained 1,000 milligrams of sodium per liter, and all the rest had water that was considerably saltier than it had been before being softened. Water softeners, you see, substitute some minerals for others. When they take out the calcium and magnesium that tend to leave rings around the bathtub, they substitute sodium.

The researchers found, furthermore, that varying amounts of sodium were left in the drinking water, depending upon how far along in the cycle of regeneration the softener was. So there would really be no way for anyone with a water softener to know how much salt he was getting in his water at any given time, for it probably varies from month to month.

The American Heart Association, in recommending diets which allow only 500 to 1,000 milligrams (½ to 1 gram) of salt per day, recommended that distilled water be used if the usual water supply contains more than 20 milligrams of sodium per liter. As we have seen, one of the homes investigated had more than 50 times that amount of salt, after the water had been softened. For the record, the average person consumes from 3 to 7 grams of salt per day, according to *Food*.

The summary of the *Archives* article states that naturally occurring well waters frequently contain concentrations of sodium that make them unsuitable for consumption by patients on salt-restricted diets. And well water treated by a cationic exchange softener almost invariably contains too much sodium for these patients.

A warning about the use of water softeners came from the City Health Commissioner of New York who, in March 1967, sent a letter to 18,000 physicians in the city reminding them that softening water increases its salt content. Therefore, patients with heart and kidney conditions that necessitate their cutting down drastically on salt may be getting as much in their daily drinking water as they are allowed for the day—without any allowance for the salt in their food. The Commissioner recommended that people with water softeners either buy bottled spring water or install their softener in such a way that unsoftened water is available for drinking and cooking. Incidentally, the label on bottled water should show the amount of sodium and other properties the water contains.

Speaking about salt, several years ago the FDA withdrew from sale vitamin C prepared from sodium ascorbate rather than ascorbic acid. There was nothing unwholesome or undesirable about the sodium ascorbate. It was vitamin C and just as effective in the body as any other kind of vitamin C. But it was the sodium part of the formula that worried the FDA. Their contention was that, if persons on a low-salt diet took this form of the vitamin in quite large doses, they might get too much sodium. Said the FDA, if these people did not look at the label, they might not know that they were getting this extra sodium.

If you are on a low-salt diet and you have a water softener, have it connected to the hot water intake only. Then be sure to use only cold water for drinking and cooking. If your municipal water supply can give you the information, ask them what the sodium content of water is in your community. If you are still not satisfied, either buy a water distiller which will remove all minerals from your drinking water, or buy bottled spring water or bottled distilled water. Distilled water is just plain H_2O with no minerals at all.

Planning a low-sodium diet is not difficult nor is it usually necessary for you to eliminate foods that are naturally rather rich in salt. What you must do, of course, is to eliminate those to which salt has been added. And you must not add any salt in the preparation of food, either in the kitchen or at the table.

Just about everything you can buy in the supermarket in the way of a prepared food contains added salt: canned soup, bread, cakes and pies, salad dressings, sauces, many canned vegetables, cheese, baloney, liver-wurst, sausage, canned meats, pickles, olives, potato chips, salted nuts. The list is almost endless.

But there is plenty of food left to eat. Meat—except for salted meats like ham, bacon and dried beef—is permissible. Fortunately eggs come in a shell, so they cannot be flavored, salted or chemicalized on the way to the table. Milk is another good choice. Yogurt is not salted. Many stores have cottage cheese that has not been salted. You can probably get unsalted butter. Fish—except for salted fish, of course—and poultry are allowed. You can eat all the fresh fruits and vegetables you want, plus unsalted nuts and dried fruits.

Frozen foods do not contain salt, unless they come with an instant sauce or gravy, or unless they are fully pre-pared dishes which you only thaw and eat. The sensible shopper avoids these so-called TV dinners anyway, because they are likely to contain added chemicals, pre-servatives, thickeners, etc. In any case, they are nutrition-ally poor for the amount you spend on them.

Oatmeal and farina, two excellent breakfast dishes, are quite low in sodium. But the prepared breakfast cereals have had considerable amounts of salt added in the processing. Buy your cereals at your health food store. Most baker's bread is loaded with salt. So are crackers, •

unless they are labeled unsalted. Why not bake your own bread?

Salad oils such as safflower oil, sunflower oil, olive oil, etc., contain almost no salt. Use them freely in place of butter, especially if you can't get unsalted butter. Use them in hearty salads at lunch and dinner. If you like onions and/or garlic, there is no limit to the amount of these excellent foods you can chop into your salads, as well as using them freely to season vegetables, breads, meat loaves and casseroles.

Herbs should become your other mainstay for flavoring salt-free dishes. Because of the recent awakening of interest in herb cookery, these tangy, flavorful and inexpensive dried leaves, seeds and flowers are readily available. Avoid prepared condiments like mustard and chilisauce—both heavily salted. On the other hand, either raw or prepared horseradish contains almost no salt but adds a zip and a tingle, especially to beef dishes. Celery and parsley, radishes and peppers are common foods that can be used much more freely. Locate a source of watercress to use in salads whenever it is available. This spicy green is rich in many valuable minerals, including iodine.

Thus, we have seen that sodium is present in most of our foods and in some of the materials we use in preparing and processing food. Ordinary table salt is 43 per cent sodium and our most concentrated source. Baking soda is about 30 per cent sodium; ordinary baking powders contain about 10 per cent, reports *Food*. A raw potato contains about 0.001 gram of sodium, but the same weight of potato chips may have as much as 0.340 gram of sodium. And cured ham has about 20 times more sodium than fresh pork. A person's intake of sodium can be limited from 1.5 to 2.5 grams daily if no salt is added at any time in preparing the food, and if no salted, pickled and cured foods are used, according to *Food*.

Getting back to potassium, ordinary diets of persons in the United States supply 1.4 to 6.5 grams of potassium per person per day. "We have no evidence that the healthy person needs to limit or otherwise control his intake of potassium," says *Food*.

However, in cases of high blood pressure and heart failure where fluid has collected, doctors sometimes give diuretics—that is, drugs that induce urination. One kind of diuretic decreases the body's supply of potassium so drastically that severe reactions can result. So doctors usually recommend that the patient drink lots of fruit juices since they are rich sources of potassium.

Today's average consumer tends to think of "fruit juices" as anything that comes on the fruit juice shelves of the supermarket. But two London physicians discovered and published in the *Lancet*, August 18, 1973, the finding that, out of 100 patients in one hospital ward, only three were drinking real fruit juices. The rest were drinking some mishmash of chemicals and sugar that looks, tastes and smells like fruit juice and is, usually, a bit less expensive.

But, as you might expect, the stuff just doesn't contain any potassium to speak of. So these sick people, guzzling glass after glass of these concoctions thought they were obeying doctors' orders. Say Dr. M. C. Bateson and A. F. Lant, "It is clear . . . that if fruit beverages are to be used as a means of adding extra potassium to the diet only real fruit juice is of value." Remember that the next time you are tempted by the gaudy labels of some of the fake juices on the supermarket shelves. Shun fake foods. A good example is an orange-type mixture that usually accompanies our astronauts into space and is heavily advertised on TV.

It's in relation to medical drugs that you may get into trouble when it comes to potassium. Two dramatic cases came to our attention recently, showing the powerful effect this mineral has on body functions and the terrible consequences when, for some reason, the body lacks potassium. In these cases the potassium depletion was brought about by drugs given for high blood pressure or hypertension.

One 65-year-old woman, being treated for very high blood pressure, was found one day paralyzed and disoriented. She did not know members of her family and spoke irrationally. Her doctor had moved and she was, for the moment, without a doctor. She was taken to the hospital, where an electrocardiogram indicated to the doctor in charge that her body had lost a great deal of potassium, due to the diuretics which her former doctor had prescribed. Body functions in which potassium is concerned were seriously damaged. She was taken off all medication and was given potassium. Within a few days she was entirely well.

In another case, a doctor had given diuretics for four years to a 60-year-old woman whose blood pressure was well controlled, but who grew weaker and more fatigued every day. Finally, her electrocardiogram showed an apparent heart attack, although she felt none of the usual symptoms—pain, breathlessness, tightness across the chest. She was told she was in very serious shape and must rest for six weeks. She was given sedatives and more diuretics; she became steadily worse. She went to another doctor, who told her there was nothing wrong with her except that her potassium balance had been completely upset. He took her off all drugs and gave her potassium supplements. She recovered within a short time. Labels on diuretics indicate the danger and warn prescribing physicians that potassium must be given along with the diuretic. If the physician overlooks this warning, disasters are likely to ensue.

It is commonplace knowledge that old people are weak. That is, their muscles do not have the strength or power of young, vigorous people. Too bad, we are apt to say. That's what happens as you get older. There's nothing to be done about it. Or is there?

In Edinburgh, two University of Glasgow scientists

Here is the Potassium Content of Some Common Foods, Along with the Sodium Content:

Foods	Sodium in 1 serving of 100 grams	Potassium in 1 serving of 100 grams
Almonds	2.0	690
Brazil nuts	0.8	650
Filberts	0.8	560
Peanuts	0.8	740
Walnuts	2.0	450
Apples	0.1	68
Apricots	0.5	440
Bananas	0.1	400
Cherries	1.0	280
Oranges	0.2	170
Peaches	0.1	180
Plums	0.1	140
Strawberries	0.7	180
Barley	3.0	160
Corn	0.4	290
Oats	2.0	340
Rice	0.8	100
Wheat	2.0	430
Beans, snap	0.3	300
Lima beans	1.0	700

Foods	Sodium in 1 serving of 100 grams	Potassium in 1 serving of 100 grams
Navy beans, dry	0.9	1,300
Fresh peas	0.9	380
Broccoli	16.0	400
Cabbage	5.0	230
Cauliflower	24.0	400
Lettuce	12.0	140
Spinach	190.0	790
Celery	110.0	300
Beets	110.0	350
Carrots	31.0	410
Potatoes	0.6	410
Turnips	5.0	260
Whole eggs	14.0	130
Whole milk	51.0	140
Beef	53.0	380
Chicken	110.0	250
Fish	60.0	360
Lamb	110.0	340
Turkey	92.0	310

tested a large number of elderly people to see how the pressure of their right-handed grip compared to that of younger people. Not surprisingly, as reported in *Medical World News*, October 6, 1969, the old folks showed up very badly in the test. But an additional observation showed that the old folks were getting very little potassium. To be exact, 60 per cent of the woman and 40 per cent of the men were not getting an adequate amount in their diets. Furthermore, Dr. Nairn R. Cowan and Dr. Thomas G. Judge found that those with the least potassium in their diets had the weakest grip and, as the potassium in the diet decreased, their muscles became progressively weaker. Said the scientists, potassium depletion (not just partial lack—but depletion) is relatively common to the elderly. Muscle strength generally declines with advancing age and potassium depletion is known to be associated with physical weakness.

As we know, all groups of foods contain ample potassium. And most foods, except for those of animal origin, contain very little sodium. See the chart on page 147. Almonds, for example contain only 2 milligrams of sodium and 690 milligrams of potassium. If almonds made up a large part of your diet—and this might be possible for some vegetarians—how is it possible that you could get too much sodium for the amount of potassium you get in almonds? It's possible because you may eat your almonds heavily dosed with salt. As long as you restrain your intake of salt—we didn't say eliminate or even sharply restrict it—just restrain that saltshaker, you're not likely to get into any trouble getting enough potassium.

We will conclude this chapter with some additional information on chlorine. A Michigan physician declares unequivocally that chlorine in drinking water is a major cause of heart attacks and other circulatory ailments. Dr. Joseph M. Price, therefore, recommends using ultraviolet light to purify city water rather than chlorine. Some of his arguments are very convincing. They are contained in a 92-page paperback, *Coronaries, Cholesterol, Chlorine* (Pyramid Books, New York City).

In his experiments, Dr. Price gave two groups of chickens exactly the same diet, but gave one group chlorinated water and another group untreated well water. The chickens which drank the chlorinated water soon began to suffer from circulatory ailments and eventually died of enlarged hearts and hemorrhages. Those which had been drinking well water showed no hardening of the arteries or abnormal hearts.

In the book, Dr. Price discusses the several reasons which orthodox medicine claims are responsible for heart attacks: too much fat and cholesterol in food, too much smoking and "stress," too much sugar and refined starches, too little exercise, etc. Then he presents his theory that a lifetime of drinking chlorinated water is responsible for our heart attack fatality figures and for our shocking incidence of other circulatory disorders. It's a provocative assumption that needs additional corroboration.

Another aspect of this theory, which Dr. Price does not mention, is that chlorine is very destructive of vitamin E. Deficiency in vitamin E has been mentioned many times as a leading cause of heart and artery diseases. Could the chlorine in drinking water be destroying that small amount of vitamin E in food, either in its preparation or its digestion?

CHAPTER 13

Copper

YOU HAVE PROBABLY never heard of copper being used for anything but wire, water pipes, jewelry, coins, etc. But this reddish-brown substance is an essential mineral for good health for all mammals. Although copper deficiency is supposedly quite uncommon in human beings, it has been observed in victims of certain disorders where absorption of food is impaired.

A review of the subject of trace minerals which appeared in *Dairy Council Digest* for July-August, 1973 tells us that study and research in the field of trace minerals is, at present, at about the same stage as vitamin research was in the late 1930's. So we have a long way to go before we discover the full story on all the trace minerals, if, indeed, we ever do. The trace mineral copper is no exception to this statement. Our scientists actually know very little about it—that is, why we need it, what it does in the body, what would occur in case of drastic deficiency and so on.

One paramount consideration seems to overpower all else in the story of copper: the copper content of the soil may determine the amount of copper in food. Plants need a certain amount of copper to grow. But food plants may contain more than that. The *Journal of the American Dietetic Association* for August, 1973 contains an article on the copper content of foods, stating that the amount of copper taken up by food plants depends on the oxidation state of the copper, the kind of copper compound it is and the acid or alkaline condition of the soil. Other considerations involve: the source of water used in irrigating or processing foods; the use of fertilizers, pesticides and fungicides.

Farmers and researchers have studied for many years the result of copper deficiency in animals which graze on copper-deficient soils. Working with laboratory animals, scientists have found that lack of copper brings about a weakness in the large heart artery, which may rupture. It seems possible that progressive increasing lack of copper over many years may play some part in the weakness of human arteries during late life. But copper deficiency, as such, resulting from lack in foods, has never been diagnosed in human beings.

Copper is involved in a number of enzyme systems in the human as well as animal body. Enzymes are proteins which sometimes have minerals as part of their structure. And enzyme systems are those processes which make things happen inside a living body. Copper helps to prevent anemia. Babies who become anemic from living too long on nothing but milk may be given iron to cure their anemia. But it is not cured unless copper is also given. Milk is short on both iron and copper.

Another function of copper is to take part in the formation of melanin, a coloring matter which influences the color of hair. As we have mentioned elsewhere in this book, in black sheep it is possible to render the animal deficient in copper and produce white wool. Returning copper to the diet, you get a band of dark wool. Taking the copper away again results in a band of white wool. The curly quality of sheep's wool is also influenced by the amount of copper in their diets. Nobody knows exactly how copper influences the color of hair and regrettably there seems to be almost no evidence that the mineral could be used to restore color to human hair that has whitened. But one cannot help but feel a nagging certainty that some day someone will discover just what combination of circumstances causes human hair to whiten and it's possible that copper may be involved.

According to *Recommended Dietary Allowances,* "Copper is an essential nutrient for all mammals. Naturally occurring or experimentally produced deficiency in animals leads to a variety of abnormalities, including anemia, skeletal defects . . . degeneration of the nervous system, defects in pigmentation and structure of hair and wool, reproductive failure and pronounced cardiovascular lesions."

Although not many cases of copper depletion have occurred in human beings, it has been found in kwashiorkor (protein starvation), sprue (a tropical disease where food is not absorbed), and the nephrotic syndrome (kidney disease).

When you get into the subject of our requirement for copper, you enter a mass of complex interrelationships among several trace minerals. E. J. Underwood, in *Trace Elements in Human and Animal Nutrition,* tells us that copper storage in the liver of animals is reduced if the animals are given more molybdenum. The amount of copper that is involved depends partly on how much sulfur there is in the diet.

It's true, too, that the amount of copper retained in the liver depends on the levels of zinc, iron and calcium carbonate in the diet. High intake of zinc means less copper and iron will be absorbed. In the body, copper concentrations are highest in liver, brain, kidneys, heart and hair. This seems to indicate that those organs need more copper than others. There is little copper in glands, a bit more in spleen, muscles, skin and bones.

This complex interrelationship of minerals is dramatically reviewed by Dr. Carl C. Pfeiffer of the New Jersey Psychiatric Institute, Stillman, New Jersey, in the December 14, 1973 issue of *Medical World News.* He tells of a patient who arrived at his clinic in 1971 suffering from "an unrelenting inferno of mental and bodily suffering."

She had suffered over the years from insomnia, loss of reality, attempted suicide, seizures or convulsions, vomiting and difficulty with menstruation. She had been given nerve tests and psychiatric tests and they were normal. She had been hospitalized and tranquilized, all to no avail. Transferring from one hospital to another, she came finally to Dr. Pfeiffer, who gave her chemical tests to determine her body's balance of nutrients—vitamins and minerals, and psychiatric tests to determine whether she suffered from perceptive disorders—that is, whether things looked peculiar to her, sounded peculiar, tasted or smelled strange.

Dr. Pfeiffer treated her with massive doses of pyridoxine (vitamin B6) and supplements of zinc and manganese. The young woman had trouble with knee joints when she began to menstruate, which gave him the clue that she might need these two minerals. And he gave her group therapy and a tranquilizer. He says that the food supplements should be given in two doses a day so that they flood the system of the patient.

The patient improved with the vitamin-mineral therapy. When it was discontinued, she relapsed. Returned to this simple therapy, she improved to such an extent that she has been free from convulsions for two years without other medication. She has made up the schooling she missed and is planning to become a doctor.

Testing urine for the presence of a "mauve factor" has become a standard test for schizophrenia among physicians and psychiatrists who use megavitamin therapy in their treatment of this severe mental illness, which disables many thousands of Americans every year. Dr. Pfeiffer says that 30 to 40 per cent of all schizophrenics excrete in their urine a certain substance which turns a deep pink or mauve when tested on a laboratory machine. The substance has been identified as something which the disordered, unbalanced body chemistry of the mentally ill person is excreting. This condition was reported in medical journals as long ago as 1963 by Dr. Abram Hoffer of Saskatoon, Canada, and Dr. Humphrey Osmond of New Jersey.

The mauve factor—or "malvaria"—seems to indicate that copper levels are normal in these people, whereas, in other schizophrenics who do not have it, copper is lacking. Other symptoms: white spots on fingernails, loss of the ability to dream or to remember dreams after waking, a distinctive, sweetish odor on the breath and abdominal pain in the left upper side of the abdomen, constipation, inability to tan in sunlight, itching in sunlight, malformation of knee cartilages, joint pains. They may also have anemia, tremor and muscle spasms. They may be impotent or have menstrual difficulties, low blood sugar and an anemia which does not respond to iron but is improved when they are given vitamin B6.

If you know someone suffering from schizophrenia, have them contact the Huxley Institute for Biosocial Research, 1114 First Ave., New York City 10021, for literature and the names and addresses of doctors, psychiatrists, clinics, etc., who may be able to help.

It is believed officially that human adults need about 2 milligrams of copper daily. Dr. Underwood believes that most people get from 2 to 4 milligrams daily. The amount of copper we get in food depends not only on the amount in the original food, but also on the amount of copper used in the processing and storing of the food. Many pesticides and fungicides include copper as an ingredient. How much of this remains in our food? Beverages processed or stored in copper containers are bound to pick up some of this trace mineral from the containers.

Dr. Underwood tells us that Dr. Henry Schroeder and his colleagues at Dartmouth have studied the progressive increase of copper in water—from a brook, to a reservoir, to a hospital tap. They also reported that there is considerably more copper in soft water than in hard water piped into homes. Some soft waters are especially effective in corroding copper from copper pipes. This might raise the copper content of the water by as much as 1.4 milligrams a day. Hard water going through the same pipes might bring in less than 0.05 milligrams a day. It seems wise always to use unsoftened water for drinking and cooking. And it seems wise to use only cold water for drinking and cooking, since copper and other minerals may be involved in the lining of the hot water heater.

There is a known relationship between copper and vitamin C. The vitamin is destroyed or oxidized in the presence of copper. Of course, inside your body this is a natural process. Vitamin C must be oxidized in order to perform its functions. But outside the body—before you eat the vitamin C—be sure it does not come in contact with copper. The copper will destroy it. These days we do not use copper on the inside of cooking utensils, mugs, dishes and bowls. But avoid using kitchen knives or spoons which may be worn and have copper linings showing.

"Wilson's disease is a genetic disorder that causes an abnormal accumulation of copper in the liver, brain, kidneys and corneas," reports *Science News*, September 29, 1973. "The disease is also characterized by an unusually high amount of copper in the bloodstream not bound to a blood protein called ceruloplasmin. Various theories have been proposed to explain the biochemical basis of Wilson's disease, but none have been proven. Now it looks as if there is at least a partial explanation— an abnormal protein in the liver. This protein can bind copper four times as well as its normal counterpart can.

"The abnormal liver protein explains some of the defects in Wilson's disease," *Science News* goes on. "A normal liver incorporates copper into enzymes or excretes copper. The abnormal protein probably causes the liver to retain copper and to decrease the incorporation of copper into ceruloplasmin. Whether the abnormal protein is also involved in the accumulation of copper in the brain, kidneys and corneas is yet to be shown."

The finding, by R. S. Dubois and K. M. Hambridge of the University of Colorado Medical Center and by G. W. Evans of the U. S. Department of Agriculture in Grand Forks, N.D., was originally reported in the September 21, 1973 issue of *Science*.

"Studies conducted at the University of Michigan suggest that students with high marks tend to have more than normal amounts of zinc and copper in their hair, but less than normal iodine," states *Fitness for Living*, September-October 1973. "The opposite appears to be true for students with low grades. Dr. Adon A. Gordus, Professor of Chemistry and director of the study, writing in *Medical Tribune,* May 9, 1973, says that other studies with rats also show a relationship between zinc and intelligence. So far, there is no evidence to link zinc intake with intelligence. It's entirely possible that those of high intelligence simply excrete more zinc."

In July 18, 1966 a curious tale appeared in *Scientific American* which was discussed in a later edition by two scientists. It seems that it was the practice, in some parts of the country long ago, to implant a penny or other copper coin under the skin of horses "to prevent some disease." Dr. Jack Schubert of the University of Pittsburgh Graduate School of Public Health remarked in a letter to the editor that sheep and cattle grazing in areas deficient in certain minerals may develop brittle bones and a condition similar to scurvy, which is the disease of vitamin C deficiency.

These changes also occur in areas where there is very high concentration of molybdenum in soil. Apparently the over-abundant amounts of molybdenum cause the animals to excrete copper, so that they become deficient in copper. He says that the horses with copper coins implanted under their skins may have lived in an area which produced a copper deficiency in them. Since their requirement for this metal is very small, they probably would have absorbed enough of it from the penny to prevent them from going lame.

The richest sources of copper in food are shellfish, especially oysters, and the organ meats like liver, kidney and brain. Nuts, seeds, legumes, raisins and prunes are good sources. Milk and other dairy products are very poor sources of either iron or copper, which emphasizes once again how wise it is to eat a wide variety of foods and not to depend on only one kind, or to get in the habit of avoiding certain nourishing foods.

Non-leafy vegetables—potatoes, carrots, etc.—contain up to 2 parts per million of copper, as do refined cereals and white bread. "The refining of cereals for human consumption," says Dr. Underwood, "results in a significant loss of copper, as with most other minerals. Thus the mean copper content of the whole grain of North American hard wheats was reported to be 5.3 parts per million, whereas the copper content of the white (72 per cent extraction) flour made from these wheats averaged only 1.7 parts per million." Thus, while we must beware of the possibility of picking up too much copper from water pipes and other contaminants, we must also be on guard against getting too little through using too many refined and processed foods, rather than wholly natural ones.

The fact that plant food may be short on copper due to methods of fertilizing emphasizes once again the importance of eating, as much as possible, organically grown food. Dr. Henry Schroeder, in *Pollution, Profits and Progress*, says that "Western man cannot bring himself to the Oriental solution of the problem: that is, putting back on the land what was taken from the land—the practice which should obtain in any true ecosystem. The best he can do is to confine his sewage to organic material which can be degraded by natural biodegradable processes, and limit the amounts to those the processes can cope with. Surpluses must be treated and restored to the land in the form of minerals which are the basic builders of life."

Two researchers from the University of California, Jean T. Pennington and Doris Howes Calloway, writing on "Copper Content of Foods" in the *Journal of the American Dietetic Association*, explain the wide variation in copper content of various foods on their list by reminding us that the copper of soils in New Jersey, for example, varies from 2 to 60 parts per million, depending on soil type and environmental contamination. As this study was done almost 10 years ago, there is little question that the contamination is far greater by now.

They also tell us that "differences due to geographic location probably result from copper contamination of water, air or soil—related to the proximity of industry and metal works—and of copper depletion due to habitual agricultural practices." This last phrase says something that organic gardeners have known for many years—that continuing, season after season, to take off crops from a given patch of soil, without replacing the valuable trace minerals, is bound to result in food deficient in the trace minerals . . . regardless of what those bureaucrats in the Food and Drug Administration may be saying.

Here is the copper content of one serving of some common foods, as outlined in the *Journal* article:

Liver, depending on what kind, from 0.11 milligram for chicken liver to 20.10 for lamb liver.
Heart, from 0.23 to 0.35 milligram.
Kidney, from 0.11 to 0.47 milligram.
Beef, up to 0.19 milligram.
Pork, up to 0.02 milligram.
Chicken, up to 0.41 milligram.
Turkey, up to 0.20 milligram.
Eggs, up to 0.23 milligram.
Fish, depending on the kind, up to 0.55 milligram.
Lobster, up to 4 milligrams.

Crab, up to 6.50 milligrams.

Oysters, up to 160 milligrams.

Cheese, up to 1.81 milligrams.

Milk, up to 0.4 milligram.

Nuts, depending on kind, up to 3.20 milligrams.

Sunflower seeds, up to 1.90 milligrams.

Sesame seeds, up to 1.59 milligrams.

Wheat bran, up to 2.66 milligrams.

Wheat germ, up to 5.17 milligrams.

Brewers yeast, up to 10.14 milligrams.

Fruits and vegetables contain considerably less copper than the foods listed above.

CHAPTER 14

Chromium

A SUBSTANCE GIVEN either as a supplement or incorporated in a food like bran or brewers yeast, which can regulate blood sugar levels, thus correcting the basic defect in diabetes, a substance which can lower cholesterol levels and, in animals, prevent a form of blindness: Is it a magic potion? Is it a newly discovered wonder vitamin?

No, it's chromium. This is a trace mineral which is mined in millions of tons for industrial consumption and which exists in the average human being in amounts as small as 1½ milligrams. It is pronounced as essential to human health by Dr. Henry Schroeder, the Dartmouth trace mineral expert, and by Dr. E. J. Underwood, both of whom are mentioned often in this book.

The official booklet of the National Academy of Sciences says of chromium, "There is some evidence that chromium is a required nutrient." We suggest that the evidence is overwhelming, and that the evidence is involved with a very special aspect of diet, nutrition and disease which is rapidly becoming of paramount importance to all human beings who live in that part of the world which we call "developed" or "industrialized."

Dr. Walter Mertz, in his testimony before the Senate Select Committee on Nutrition and Human Needs, April 30, 1973, said: "Another element we are concerned about is chromium. Here, as with other elements, the numbers of subjects examined are not enough to make a sweeping statement. We do know that chromium deficiency exists in countries with protein nutrition problems, but that it also exists in part of our older population, as evidenced by the fact that we can improve the impaired glucose tolerance in about 50 per cent of the subjects examined by increasing their chromium intake."

As we have said, chromium appears to be intimately related to the way the body uses sugar—all kinds of sugars: glucose (the stuff the doctor gives you to drink when he's testing your blood sugar), white sugar, brown sugar, dark brown sugar, molasses and—of all things—brewers yeast.

Dr. Underwood tells us that as long ago as 1957 two researchers discovered that laboratory rats on a deficient diet developed "impaired glucose tolerance," which means that their blood sugar regulating mechanisms were unable to deal with starches and sugars. They tended to become diabetic. These researchers decided they had found a new dietary agent which they called GTF (glucose tolerance factor). Later investigation revealed that this factor was chromium. Giving regulated amounts of chromium, the scientists could successfully restore proper blood sugar regulation, thus preventing diabetes. Then they found that certain chemical forms of the mineral did not accomplish the desired object, but that, when they gave brewers yeast, they seemed to be giving the real GTF which they decided must be a chromium-containing complex of things.

Dr. Schroeder, working at Dartmouth in a laboratory where any contamination with trace minerals is impossible, tested rats on a diet in which there was almost no chromium. The rats developed "moderate diabetes mellitus." It was rapidly reversed when the scientists gave the rats several parts per million of chromium in their drinking water.

Later in a controlled trial, 3 of 6 mild diabetics were given chromium and showed significant improvement in their condition. Two more patients showed some improvement, while one more did not. In a study of old people with diabetes, 10 were given chromium supplements for 2 to 3 months. Four of these improved to such an extent that their blood sugar tests were normal. The remaining six did not benefit. "This suggests," says Dr. Underwood, "that the low chromium state of the responding patients had not yet been complicated by other factors."

Other facts began to come in. In Africa and the Near East hungry children were shown to have disordered blood sugar levels. Giving them chromium improved them "spectacularly" within 18 hours. Other studies showed that, in locations where there was plenty of chromium in the drinking water, there were not so many cases of blood sugar disorder.

More recently, a physician in a Birmingham, Alabama hospital did a study on the chromium content in the livers of three groups of patients. Those with high blood pressure and hardening of the arteries had seemingly plenty of chromium in their livers. The third group were diabetics, and only in this group was the chromium content low, in comparison with a control group of healthy persons. This seems to indicate that the diabetic is either unable to use chromium properly or that he does not get enough of it in his food.

In *Nutrition Reviews*, February, 1967, we learn that chromium, given to people who had diabetic tendencies, appeared to improve their blood sugar conditions. The mineral itself does not seem to cause blood sugar levels to decrease, we are told, but it may in some way make the action of insulin more effective. The author points out that this mineral seems to decrease in human bodies as we grow older. One wonders, he says, whether the tendency toward a progressive decrease in body chromium contributes to the higher incidence of diabetes mellitus and degenerative vascular disease in older people.

Diabetes, August, 1968, reported a test of the hair of a group of diabetic children compared with that of normal children. For 19 children with diabetes, the chromium content of the hair averaged about 0.55 milligrams per gram. For 33 normal children, the chromium content averaged about 0.85 milligrams per gram, reports Dr. R. A. Kreisberg. One of the conditions almost always associated with diabetes—if the disease continues uncontrolled—is raised cholesterol levels of blood, which can lead to all kinds of circulatory troubles. So one scientist decided to add chromium to a low-chromium diet and see what this did to cholesterol levels. It lowered them, without any other changes in the diet.

Dr. Schroeder tried the same experiment at Dartmouth using rats on diets in which different sugars were used. The blood levels of cholesterol were higher and increased with age in rats which got white sugar, which is very low in chromium. Those which were getting brown sugar, or white sugar plus chromium, had low levels of cholesterol. When one considers that these experiments were conducted and reported in 1969, there seems to be almost no excuse for continuing propaganda which incessantly tells us that people have high cholesterol levels because they eat too many eggs.

In *Pollution, Profits and Progress*, Dr. Schroeder tells us that, when we refine sugar from sugarcane to make white sugar, we remove 94 per cent of the chromium. When we remove the bran and germ of wheat to make white flour and processed cereals, we remove 50 per cent of the chromium, along with, of course, many other trace minerals. To make up for these losses, we then put some iron in the flour or cereals and call them "enriched."

"Little is known of the chemical forms in which chromium exists in food plants," says Dr. Underwood. In other words, biochemists do not know, as yet, how to give anybody the same form of chromium that exists in food because they just don't know what form that may be. If they give the mineral in some form that can't be easily absorbed by the body, results will not be good. However, says Dr. Underwood, "Foods rich in GTF—such as brewers yeast—are, therefore, quantitatively superior, per unit of chromium, to others with less of their chromium in this form," and superior, too, to simple salts of chromium, which is the kind the doctor might give you.

"Chromium resembles most trace minerals in being concentrated in the branny layers and the germ of cereal grains," says Dr. Underwood. One sample of whole wheat contained 1.7 parts per million of chromium, compared with only 0.23 parts in a white flour and 0.14 parts per million in a loaf of white bread. Brown and raw sugars contain considerable amounts of this mineral in comparison with white sugar.

The amount of chromium any human being gets is greatly influenced, therefore, by the amount of refined carbohydrates he eats. A scientist who studied an institutional diet (a hospital or a school, we suppose) found about 80 micrograms of chromium per person per day in the food. The diabetic old people we referred to earlier, some of whom had a dramatic response to chromium, were getting only about 50 micrograms of the trace mineral per day in their food. Another study of two adults who were not diabetic showed that they were getting 330 and 400 micrograms per day.

In the *American Journal of Clinical Nutrition*, March, 1968, Dr. Schroeder reports on animal experiments that were conducted 10 years before. In one experiment, arteries of rats fed various diets were examined after their deaths. 19 per cent of those on diets deficient in chromium showed fatty deposits in the artery that leads to the heart. Only 2 per cent of those getting enough chromium had these possibly dangerous deposits.

Dr. Schroeder has also carefully examined records of the amount of chromium in various organs of Americans, compared to that found in organs of people in the Near and Far East. In every case, the Americans have far lower levels. For instance, men from 20 to 59 years of age were examined in one survey. The amount of chromium in the important heart artery of Americans averaged only 1.9 parts per million, while African men had 5.5, Near Eastern men had 11 and men from the Far East had 15 ppm. In the brain, heart, kidneys, liver, pancreas, etc., similar conditions were found. It has also been found that the organs of wild animals contain far more chromium than those of modern Americans.

Dr. Underwood and Dr. Schroeder tell us that there are great differences among various drinking waters in this country in regard to the amount of chromium they contain, some having three times as much as others.

What about blindness? There is not much evidence available on this subject, but *Nutrition Reviews*, July 1968, reported on a study done in 1967 which involved laboratory rats fed a diet which was adequate in all nutrients except chromium. Half the group ate this diet permanently. No chromium was available in either water or food. A second group ate the same diet but had drinking water which contained 2 parts per million of chromium. Within two to three weeks the rats which got no chromium began to show deterioration of part of the cornea. Ten of the 60 rats ultimately developed corneal opacity, which would presumably lead to blindness. No opacities developed in the rats which got the chromium supplement.

Before you write to ask us, let us say that we cannot state categorically that getting plenty of chromium in your diet will prevent or cure diabetes. Also, we do not know at the present time where you can get chromium salts to take if you want to try to prevent diabetes. Perhaps your doctor can read up on this subject and discover a source. What we can tell you is very much what Dr. Henry Schroeder says in his book, as follows:

"Arteriosclerosis or hardening of the arteries can be duplicated in the monkey by vitamin B6 deficiency and in the rat by chromium deficiency. Practically everyone in the United States gets this disease and half of us die of it. Most Americans are chromium deficient, largely because we eat foods from which chromium has been removed by refining. The natural form of chromium in foods is not known—but soon will be. This form regulates our efficiency in using sugar and fat and in keeping cholesterol under control. When it is available, we will be able to prevent, if not cure, this fatal disease. Until then the best we can do is to avoid the white of Purity, and stick to dark brown sugar, whole wheat bread, natural fat, whole grains and cereals and nuts, which have plenty of chromium. Bran is loaded with it. And we certainly should take extra vitamin B6 (pyridoxine)."

And, we would add, use plenty of brewers yeast.

CHAPTER 15

Cobalt

IN ONE OF the most crazy, mixed-up detective stories of all nutritional science, it was discovered in 1948 that the nutritional factor which could cure pernicious anemia in human beings was a compound containing the trace mineral cobalt. Since 1935 scientists had been perplexed by a disease of sheep and cattle in Australia called "coast disease" or "wasting disease." They discovered that the disease was caused by lack of cobalt in the soil, hence in the food the animals were eating. Cobalt is a silver-white metallic substance with a faint pink tinge; it occurs in silicates, which afford blue coloring substances for ceramics.

Researchers gave the sick animals cobalt supplements and the disease was cured. Such detective work takes time, money and facilities—and it's far more exciting, in its way, than the kind of detective stories we read or watch on TV.

So how is the soil deficiency in cobalt related to pernicious anemia? Another detective story. Scientists thought that vitamin B12—which can cure pernicious anemia—might be the functional form of cobalt in animals which eat and digest their food as sheep and cattle do—the ruminant animals, that is. The next time cobalt deficiency caused the "wasting disease" in lambs, they injected the lambs with vitamin B12 and cured the affliction. Apparently the animals were unable to synthesize enough vitamin B12 to keep themselves healthy when they weren't getting enough cobalt in their food.

Containing perhaps the most complex chemical formula of any vitamin, B12 is the only vitamin to contain a metal—cobalt—and also phosphorus. Unlike many vitamins, B12 cannot be duplicated synthetically in a laboratory. It is, therefore, the most potent of known vitamins. The daily human requirements amount to only a few micrograms.

There is no evidence of cobalt deficiency in human beings, even in parts of the world where there is not enough cobalt in the soil to keep ruminant animals healthy. "The significance of cobalt in human health and nutrition is confined, so far as is now known, to its rare presence in vitamin B12," says Dr. Underwood. "All ordinary diets supply much more cobalt than can be accounted for as vitamin B12 and no relationship necessarily exists between their cobalt and their vitamin B12 contents."

Two Russian scientists reported in a Russian journal in 1971 that sizable amounts of copper and cobalt were concentrated in bran, while the whiter the flour made from wholegrains, the less of all the trace minerals it contained. This finding seems to run consistently through all research in regard to trace minerals. Surely the old adage "the whiter the bread, the sooner you're dead" is more than confirmed by modern trace mineral research.

Green leafy vegetables contain more cobalt than other foods, with dairy products and refined cereals the poorest sources. Vitamin B12 is found chiefly in products of animal source: liver, meat, eggs.

CHAPTER 16

Manganese

MANGANESE IS A trace element known to be essential for good health, but no one has ever seen a deficiency in human beings, according to official statements by the National Academy of Sciences. Thus, no official level has been set for a recommended dietary allowance.

According to other researchers, however, it seems that this rather mysterious mineral plays a very important part in some activities inside the human body which become especially interesting in "developed," highly industrialized countries where refined carbohydrates make up such a large part of the diet—almost one-half of everything that most Americans eat, according to some estimates. Like chromium, manganese is involved in those body functions that evolve around sugar and starch. And like chromium, manganese is removed almost entirely when starchy foods like flour and cereals are refined and when sugar is refined from sugar cane or sugar beets.

Dr. Henry Schroeder tells us, in *Pollution, Profits and Progress,* that United States industry uses about 2 million tons of manganese every year. Everyone of us has a total of about 12 milligrams of manganese inside us. We get it from food and drinking water. Much of this amount is tied up in bone structure. Animals which do not get enough manganese develop dreadful bone symptoms: lameness, shortened, crooked legs, enlarged hocks, retarded bone growth, deformities, twisting and bending of bones and joints. Chickens especially suffer from a condition called perosis, which cripples and eventually kills them. Another condition brought about by lack of this mineral in the diet is called nutritional chrondrodystrophy, which deforms their jaws and heads and usually kills them. Rats, rabbits, pigs, lambs and many other animals suffer serious difficulties of this kind when their feeds do not contain enough manganese.

Lack of the mineral also affects eggs and their shells. The strength of the shell and the mineral content of the egg are determined in part by the amount of manganese in the hen's feed. In chicks and baby animals alike, deformities result in the young when the mother is not getting enough manganese.

We know very little about this mineral in relation to human health. We do know that stores of it are found chiefly in the human liver, kidney, pancreas, lungs, prostate gland, adrenals and brain, as well as bone. We also know that, following severe heart attacks, levels of manganese are raised in the blood. In fact, doctors sometimes diagnose heart attacks by measuring the amount of this mineral in the blood of the patient. We know, too, that the red blood cells of people with rheumatoid arthritis contain more manganese than normal, although we do not as yet know why.

Manganese is part of certain important enzyme systems, including one which is responsible for the formation of urea in the body. We know also that the body has a very effective method for regulating the amounts of this mineral that will remain in the body. There is no problem of getting too much, as is the case with sodium or fluoride. The body simply regulates its supply and excretes whatever is not being used.

In 1968, two scientists definitely established that manganese is closely involved in the way our bodies use sugar. Using guinea pigs that had been made deficient in the mineral, scientists gave them sugar and found that they reacted like diabetics. Their pancreatic glands were unable to handle the load of sugar and it spilled over into the urine, after raising the blood sugar higher than it should be. Giving the animals manganese completely reversed this process and brought about a normal reaction.

By 1962, doctors were giving manganese to their diabetic patients and getting a healthy reduction in blood sugar. Other doctors were finding that, when they removed the pancreas gland or when a patient contracted diabetes, the manganese in his blood decreased. We do not know at this point whether the mineral is involved in manufacturing the hormone insulin, which, as we know, regulates blood sugar levels. But it does seem possible. It also seems possible that it may be useful in other ways for regulating blood sugar levels.

The December 29, 1962 issue of *Lancet* describes a young man who was brought into the Johannesburg General Hospital in South Africa in a diabetic coma. He had been a diabetic for seven years and suffered from inability to control the wild swings from high to low blood sugar. He had been hospitalized many times, usually for the same reason—his blood sugar was too low. The doctors tried to treat him with insulin, but the 18-year-old responded badly. His blood sugar level had reached 648 milligrams per 100 ml—a fantastically high figure—when he mentioned that he had been using an ancient folk medicine (alfalfa tea) to control his diabetes.

The doctors were desperate so they told him to make some of the tea there in the ward. He boiled alfalfa leaves, made an infusion and drank it. The doctors watched and tested. Within two hours, his blood sugar level fell to 68 milligrams. Twelve times in the next weeks they gave the boy alfalfa tea and 12 times his soaring blood sugar fell rapidly. They tried the experiment at different times of the day and at different intervals after meals. The results were always happily the same.

One of the doctors remembered that alfalfa contains considerable amounts of manganese. They gave the boy a measured amount of manganese and the same reaction took place—blood sugar dropped dramatically and rapidly. The boy was released from the hospital, but, since he did not take his drug at the proper time, neglected his diet, and eventually became violent and dangerous, he was readmitted. This time, the doctors removed part of his pancreas and later found that they could control his diabetes with insulin.

The doctors conclude their article by theorizing that the action of the manganese in the alfalfa tea must mean that the patient was deficient in this mineral. Since he had no dietary deficiency and since the amount needed is very small, it seemed to them that something in his make-up was rendering the manganese unavailable to him.

How is it possible that any human being could become deficient in this mineral which is apparently quite widespread in nature? Easy. There are widespread soil deficiencies so far as manganese is concerned, according to Dr. Underwood in *Trace Elements in Human and Animal Nutrition*. And there are big differences in the amount of this mineral in drinking water sources throughout the country.

Then there are differences in the amount of manganese found in different foods that are staples. Corn is deficient in this mineral. Wheat and oats contain the most manganese of all cereals, barley a bit less. So people who depend almost entirely on corn as their basic cereal may be suffering from low amounts of manganese in their diets. Adding wheat bran would easily correct this condition, since bran is one of the richest sources of manganese.

Says Dr. Underwood, "The wide range for manganese in cereal grains and their products is due partly to plant species differences and partly to the effects of the milling processes which separate the manganese-rich from the manganese-poor parts of the grain. When whole wheat containing 31 parts per million of manganese was milled, it yielded 160 parts per million (of the mineral) in the germ, 119 parts per million in the bran and only 5 parts per million in low-grade flour."

Wholewheat flours average 46 parts per million of manganese, while white flours contain only about 6.5 parts per million. So, reports Dr. Underwood, the amount of manganese which any human being gets depends largely on how much unrefined cereal he gets and how much green leafy vegetables he consumes.

Tea also contains goodly amounts of manganese. Testing some British people who were known to drink a lot of tea but whose diets contained only refined cereals, no wholegrain ones, researchers found that their daily meals contained only up to 2.7 milligrams of manganese, while people who were eating a very similar diet but with wholegrain cereals and bread were getting as much as 8.8 milligrams of this mineral. So even the manganese in their tea did not make up any considerable supply of manganese for the white bread-white cereal, white-sugar eaters.

"Diets high in milk, sugar and refined cereals and low in fruits and vegetables could contain less than 5 parts per million of manganese," says Dr. Underwood. "The possibility that such diets supply insufficient manganese cannot be excluded. This possibility certainly warrants investigation with growing children and pregnant women, in view of the special involvement of manganese in skeletal development in embryonic and early life and in the reproductive processes."

He reminds us that Dr. Schroeder has suggested that the following disorders be investigated from the standpoint of possible manganese deficiency: any pregnancy conditions involving nervous instability and convulsions; bone and cartilage disorders in infants and children and certain types of sterility in both males and females. And, of course, diabetes.

We would add that the diet outlined above (milk, sugar, corn flakes and other refined cereals and almost no fresh fruits and vegetables) is precisely the diet we are told many of our old people subsist on because of lack of money, lack of interest in preparing food, lack of transportation facilities to do much shopping for more nutritious food. Could this not have an important bearing on the fact that diabetes as an accompaniment of old age is becoming almost as common as stiff joints, weak eyes and ears, lack of stamina and the other infirmities of old age?

How can we prevent these conditions in pregnant women, infants, children and old people? These are the people most likely to suffer nutritional deficiencies in our society. Well, a daily ration of wheat germ and/or bran would work near-magic, it seems, since these foods are rich in many vitamins and minerals—vitamins B1, B2, B3, B6, B12, E, inositol, folic acid, choline, pantothenic acid; minerals—iron, phosphorus, magnesium, sodium, manganese, etc. And, of course, they contain protein, carbohydrates and fat.

We cannot help but point out, in this connection, that we are being told a bare-faced lie—by Washington bureaucrats and self-styled nutrition experts who write syndicated columns—when we are told that "enriched" bread and cereals are just as good as the wholegrain variety because the food elements taken out in the refining process have all been restored in the "enrichment."

Manganese is one of the minerals that is almost entirely removed (89 per cent of it is removed from white sugar, 86 per cent from white flour). It is never replaced. Now, obviously, since it accompanies starches and sugars in foods, it is needed by the body to help process these carbohydrates. If it has been almost completely removed, how can one avoid suffering serious consequences in regard to sugar and starch? Diabetes is only one of the disorders that are part of such an out-of-kilter mechanism. There is now considerable evidence that heart and circulatory conditions may be part of the same imbalance.

What foods contain the most manganese? Those foods in the seed family which are so rich in other minerals: nuts; wholegrain cereals and products made from them; green leafy vegetables (spinach, salad greens, parsley, broccoli); fresh fruits; root vegetables (potatoes, carrots, etc.)

Nuts may contain up to 42 parts per million of manganese. Cereal products may contain up to 91 ppm. Dried legumes (beans and peas) may contain up to 28 ppm. Green leafy vegetables may contain up to 13 ppm. Dried fruits may contain up to 6.7 ppm. Fresh fruits may contain up to 10.7 ppm of manganese.

CHAPTER 17

Molybdenum

SCIENTISTS HAVE BEEN investigating molybdenum since the 1930's, when animals in one part of England were sickening from a disease called "teart," which resulted from too much molybdenum in their forage. Veterinarians treated it by giving the animals copper supplements. Australian researchers next found that giving molybdenum supplements to animals poisoned by too much copper brought improvement.

In 1953, it was discovered that this element plays a part in one enzyme, so it is assumed to be essential for many kinds of animals and birds. But, says Dr. Underwood, in *Trace Elements in Human and Animal Nutrition,* "there is little evidence that molybdenum plays any significant role in any aspect of human health or disease."

Dr. Underwood goes on to say that this mineral is apparently of so little practical significance to human nutrition that few researchers have studied it. However, according to *The New York Times,* September 29, 1972, worldwide changes in the incidence of cancers of the digestive tract are pointing to meats, alcohol and a deficiency of molybdenum in the diet as possible causes of these major cancer killers.

Dr. H. Marvin Pollard, gastroenterologist from the University of Michigan, said that, although cancer of the stomach has been on the decline among Americans, the rate of cancer of the colon and rectum (a leading killer that strikes 76,000 persons a year), is expected to increase 25 per cent by the year 2000. Cancer of the pancreas may increase 180 per cent, he believes.

Even sharper changes in cancer incidence have occurred among Black Americans, who in the last generation have experienced a tripling of cancer of the esophagus, the article states. Esophageal cancer has also increased at epidemic rates in the Transkei in South Africa, Curacao and the Caspian Peninsula in Iran, according to Dr. John W. Berg, epidemiologist at the National Cancer Institute. These remarks were addressed to the 7th National Cancer Conference, held in September, 1972 in Los Angeles.

"In the Transkei, researchers found that plants were highly deficient in the trace element molybdenum. And in the U.S., analyses of water supplies and cancer incidence data indicated that areas deficient in molybdenum also had high rates of esophageal cancer," the *Times* says.

Some of the bowel cancers may be attributed to something used in meats, Dr. Berg says. Therefore, studies are now being conducted among vegetarians, who eat no meat, and Seventh-Day Adventists, who eat little meat, to seek further confirmation of this finding.

Supposedly we get about 100 micrograms of molybdenum a day in the "average diet." A high-protein diet appears essential for the elimination of unnecessary molybdenum from the body. Legumes (beans, peas, soybeans), wholegrain cereals, leafy vegetables, liver and kidney are the best sources of this element, with fruits, root and stem vegetables, muscle meats and dairy products among the poorest.

Wheat in the United States may contain an average of about 48 parts per million of molybdenum, while white flour contains only about half this much. In other words, it's the same story as with almost all other trace minerals.

CHAPTER 18

Selenium

CORNELL UNIVERSITY RESEARCHERS have been investigating the relation of vitamin E to selenium, a trace mineral. This matter has brought much confusion to the subject of vitamin E. We know that the two elements are related and that the relationship is about as complicated as any that scientists are trying to unravel.

Milton L. Scott of Cornell has now reported that we are a step farther along the line toward understanding the puzzle. We know that vitamin E and selenium are both essential for normal growth and health of chickens and other animals, but we do not know exactly how they function. Chickens who are not getting enough of either one or the other, or both, are subject to a disease called *exudative diathesis*, which is an ailment involving swelling due to abnormal collection of body fluid under the skin. Losses of the poultry industry due to this disease run into millions of dollars annually.

On April 27, 1973, the FDA proposed the addition of limited amounts of selenium to some animal feeds. Selenium deficiency in animals can result in decreased rates of growth, disease and death, the FDA said. The Agency's proposal would allow the addition of 0.1 ppm of selenium in the feed of swine and growing chickens and 0.2 ppm in the feed of turkeys. These essentially trace amounts will satisfy nutritional requirements without causing significant increase in the selenium concentration of edible tissues of chickens, turkeys or swine, the

FDA states. Tests have shown that animals absorb dietary selenium according to bodily need and rapidly excrete any excess, the agency adds.

At a time when the FDA broadcasts far and wide that the soil has nothing to do with the mineral content of the food grown there, it is interesting to read their statement on selenium. "Levels naturally found in animal feed vary widely depending on the soil in which the feed crops were grown," the FDA states in its April 27 press release. "A recent survey of feed corn revealed that selenium content ranged from a low of 0.01 parts per million to 2.03 ppm. It is estimated that 70 per cent of the domestic corn and soybeans used for animal feed does not have adequate selenium to meet the animals' nutritional needs."

Recently work at the University of Wisconsin revealed that selenium is a basic ingredient of an enzyme in the red blood cells of rats. Herein lies the secret of selenium, apparently. Chicks which get enough selenium have a high level of this enzyme. But it drops almost to zero only five days after they are fed a diet deficient in selenium. Said Dr. Scott at a meeting of the American Societies for Experimental Biology, selenium, acting as part of this enzyme, destroys certain unhealthy by-products of fatty substances in the blood. These substances are destructive of the walls of capillaries, the smallest of the blood vessels. Selenium destroys the harmful substances after they have appeared. It now seems that one of the roles of vitamin E is to *prevent* these fatty substances from forming. So the vitamin and the trace mineral work together—the vitamin prevents the harmful substances from forming. If not enough of the vitamin is present to do this job, the trace mineral takes over and destroys the fatty byproducts that have formed.

This sounds terribly complex to a non-chemist, but it demonstrates clearly the great complexity of the things that go on inside our bodies. In this case, getting enough vitamin E gives protection. But, if the diet lacks vitamin E, the selenium can be depended upon to stop the next step toward ill-health. If both are lacking in the diet, disaster results, at least in the case of chicks. It may be years before researchers get around to discovering whether or not this same mechanism works in human beings, and still longer until we get an official recommendation that our diets include selenium, in small quantities, and vitamin E in large enough amounts to protect us.

"Large enough amounts" may be the key words here, for, as Dr. Hugh Sinclair points out in the *Lancet* (September 1, 1973), the reason for our deficiency in vitamin E is the almost complete removal of this vitamin from whole grains and the further destruction of the remnants left when chlorine is used to bleach flour so that it is easier for the bakers to work with. Vitamin E protects the unsaturated fats in the body, says Dr. Sinclair, one of England's most distinguished biologists. Vitamin E is an antioxidant. That is, it prevents the action of oxygen on the unsaturated fats, which prevents rancidity or the formation of substances called lipid peroxides.

Dr. Sinclair believes that the reason why modern men are much more susceptible to heart attacks than women is because they need more of the unsaturated fats than women need. We have already discussed how the unsaturated fats are diminished by refining. It is also true that, when unsaturated fats and oils are hardened to make commercial shortening and margarine, the unsaturated fats are destroyed. This is one reason not to use the commercial shortening and ordinary margarine. Stick with the special margarines which have been manufactured especially to retain all the unsaturated fats.

Dr. Sinclair also tells us that excess sugar is turned

into saturated fat in the body. For good health we need a balance between unsaturated and saturated fats. If, by refining flour and cereals, we destroy the unsaturated fats, then eat lots of sugar which increases the saturated fats in our bodies—we are destroying our health in two ways.

In *Nutrition Today* (July/August 1973), Dr. A. L. Tappel, Professor of Food Science and Technology and Professor of Nutrition at the University of California, tells the story of vitamin E in these terms: scientists just don't know what it does in the body except to prevent oxidation of the saturated fats. We know that it is essential for human health, he goes on, but it seems that all of us are getting plenty of the vitamin in our everyday diets, so no one ever needs more than that.

Then he contradicts himself repeatedly by pointing out that refining and bleaching flour destroys vitamin E. It's true, too, he admits, that people who have trouble absorbing fats from their digestive tracts are likely to be short on vitamin E, since it is fat-soluble. And it's true, he concedes, that vitamin E does protect animals from getting cancer from the pollutants in urban air. This kind of air pollution is admittedly recent in origin, and, perhaps, he admits, it's possible that human beings need more vitamin E to help to protect them against these recent pollutants.

It's also true, he says, that vitamin E has been shown to be very effective in treating a circulatory condition called *intermittent claudication*, which makes walking impossible for people with this condition, because of the pain it causes. He does not explain why and how a vitamin which can so easily treat this kind of circulatory condition may not be just as effective in treating other circulatory ailments—in massive doses. It's true, too, he says, that babies with a certain kind of anemia need vitamin E supplements for the sake of their red blood cells. More than 400 papers on vitamin E were published

Low Selenium Area	High Selenium Area
Chicago, Ill.	Los Angeles, Calif.
Bridgeport, Conn.	Atlanta, Ga.
Cincinnati, Ohio	San Diego, Calif.
Fall River, Mass.	Fort Worth, Texas
Providence, R. I.	Dallas, Texas
Youngstown, Ohio	Oklahoma City, Okla.
Dayton, Ohio	Phoenix, Ariz.
Albany, N. Y.	Denver, Colo.
Worcester, Mass.	Houston, Texas
Rochester, N. Y.	New Orleans, La.
Allentown, Pa.	San Antonio, Texas
Brocton, Mass.	Salt Lake City, Utah
Gary, Ind.	Tulsa, Okla.
Utica, N. Y.	Birmingham, Ala.
Toledo, Ohio	Omaha, Nebr.
Wilmington, Del.	Wichita, Kans.

in medical literature in the past year alone. But Dr. Tappel discounts all those which he prefers not to believe, calling them "badly designed experiments."

Getting back to selenium, it is also famous as a devastatingly toxic mineral under certain circumstances. It has been found to cause cancer in rats. Should we then make every effort to avoid selenium? Not at all, for the latest investigation reported on this engrossing subject indicates that selenium appears to prevent certain kinds of cancer in human beings: A paragon of paradoxes!

Two researchers associated with the Cleveland Clinic Foundation and the Cleveland Clinic Educational Foundation have done a study of the cancer incidence rates in 34 American cities, comparing those with low selenium to those with high selenium in the soil.

They found that cancer incidence is not nearly so great where there is plenty of selenium in the soil. According to Medical Tribune (June 27, 1973), where the report appeared, a low selenium area is one where the grass which forage animals eat contains up to 0.05 ppm. A medium selenium area has concentrations up to 0.10 ppm, and a high area has up to 0.11 ppm of selenium.

The Cleveland researchers investigated the soil in the cities in the chart at left.

It also seems that the amount of selenium in the diet has something to do with where in the body the cancer occurs. In cities with reduced incidence of cancer there was reduction in cancers of all parts of the digestive tract: pharynx, esophagus, small intestine, stomach, large intestine, rectum, bladder, urinary organs and kidneys.

How might selenium bring about such a reduction in cancer incidence, if these findings prove that it does? Dr. Raymond J. Shumberger tells us we know that antioxidants prevent cancer by "decreasing peroxidation that may enhance the attachment of the carcinogen to desoxyribonucleic acid," meaning that the substance which is an antioxidant prevents oxygen from reacting with other substances, hence may prevent the cancer-causing substances from attaching themselves to an extremely important substance in the cell called DNA. Dr. Shumberger states that antioxidants such as vitamin E, selenium, BHT (a preservative used in cereals) and vitamin C seem to behave this way.

Since 1939, he says, we have been adding antioxidants to commercial cereal foods. Perhaps this may explain the decrease in stomach cancers during those years. Those antioxidant substances listed above would be digested in the stomach or small intestine, thus they would not be present in the lower part of the digestive tract to give protection there. However, he said, selenium seems to protect the entire digestive tract from cancer.

Does all this mean that, if you live in or near one of the cities in the left-hand column above, you should expect to get cancer, and if you live in one of the cities on the right you should feel perfectly safe? Not at all. It does mean that, apparently, selenium—along with vitamins E and C—exercises a certain restraining effect on cancer production, which we do not as yet fully understand. But it would be wise to make certain you are not short on either of these vitamins or selenium—at mealtime and in food supplements.

How much selenium do human beings need and where can they get it? No one knows the answer to the first part of this question. The answer to the second part is that selenium occurs in those same natural foods in which other trace minerals are found: cereals, nuts, vegetables, fruits, and also in milk and meat—especially the organ meats. We have no figures on the differences between wholegrain and refined cereals, but it seems probable that the selenium is removed in the refining process, as we have often indicated in this book.

Is it possible to take a selenium pill—the kind given to animals to make up for what is not in their forage? No, because we do not as yet know that much about the selenium requirements for humans and, presumably, our scientists cannot take the chances with human lives that they take with animals. It's safe to say, however, that, if you are getting whole, natural supplements and foods which are rich in other trace minerals, the chances are that selenium will be present in ample amounts.

CHAPTER 19

Lithium

ON JUNE 22, 1973 theatrical producer and director Josh Logan appeared on the "Today" show on television with an amazing story. One of the American theater's brightest and most creative artists, Logan told a story of a lifelong struggle with what psychiatrists call the "Manic-Depressive Syndrome." A period of elation in which he was at the top of the world, talking wildly, working feverishly, doing all kinds of crazy things in a loud, uncontrolled spirit of gaiety, followed, after a few months, by a period of depression so severe that suicide seemed the only answer.

Logan described his lifelong search for a cure. He underwent just about every therapy known, all to no avail. Then he heard of a psychiatrist who was using a fairly new treatment—a pill containing one of the earth's elements, lithium. He took the pill. He appeared on "Today" with Dr. Ronald R. Fieve to demonstrate to all other sufferers from this emotional ailment that there is hope. And the hope may reside in the pill, which he will have to take all his life, just as diabetics must take insulin.

His depression is gone, his wild swings from elation to depression are a thing of the past. He no longer has "ups" in which he does hysterical things of which he is later ashamed. He no longer suffers from depression; he no longer contemplates suicide.

"I have found that some of the most gifted individuals

in our society suffer from (manic-depressive) illness," said Dr. Fieve before an American Medical Association meeting in June 1973, "including many outstanding writers, politicians, business executives and scientists— where tremendous amounts of manic energy and imagination have enabled them to achieve their heights of success." Without proper treatment, he went on, these same people "suddenly crash into a devastating depression that we only hear about after a successful suicide."

Some of the symptoms of the mania stage of this disease are excessive telephoning and talking, hyperactivity, decreased need for sleep and abnormal elation. The victim goes on shopping sprees, invests money wildly, behaves flamboyantly, grandiosely or perhaps angrily. In the depressive stage of illness, he wishes only to die. Dr. Fieve is chief of staff of the New York State Psychiatric Institute's lithium clinic and metabolic unit. He has been working with the mineral since 1959. More women than men suffer regularly from depression, says Dr. Fieve. The disorder appears to be genetically determined—that is, inherited. The disease is quite likely to be diagnosed incorrectly.

Dr. Fieve has urged the FDA to authorize the use of lithium as a preventive measure as well as a treatment. He also charged that the slow progress being made by psychiatrists using lithium is "in no small measure due to the indifference of the American pharmaceutical industry, which could hardly get excited about a simple, nonpatentable salt, offering no proprietary benefits." In other words, since the drug companies can't make any money out of selling lithium, they will not bother to investigate or promote it. The "drug," as doctors call it, was cleared by the FDA for use in the treatment of depression in 1970.

In a lengthy article—"Depression, the Common Cold of Mental Ailments"—by Rona Cherry and Laurence Cherry, in *The New York Times Magazine,* November

25, 1973, Dr. Fieve says: "There are people who have a certain vulnerability in competitive situations. They tend to give up and accept being secondary instead of fighting back—the subdued, sensitive kind of person. Now are they that way because of upbringing or heredity or both? I certainly think people have overlooked the genetic factor in all kinds of depression."

The ancient Greeks knew about lithium and knew about its powers for calming the turbulent spirit. A 5th century Greek physician recommended waters from a spring containing lithium for treating mental disturbances. The mineral was also used in the 19th century for treating gout, rheumatism and kidney stones. But lithium seems to have an upsetting effect on the sodium-potassium balance of the body. As we learned in previous chapters, these two minerals must be maintained in a certain equilibrium, since one is concentrated outside of cell walls and the other inside cell walls. Upsetting the balance can bring about swelling and kidney troubles as well as disastrous circulatory changes.

So the early work with lithium treatment was abandoned. In the 1940's drug researchers, looking for a salt substitute, hit on lithium as a flavor enhancer which could substitute for table salt. The aforementioned problems with sodium balance cut short this experiment as several people using lithium as a salt substitute died.

In 1949, an Australian psychiatrist, experimenting with animals, rediscovered lithium's calming properties and began to use it successfully on his mental patients suffering from mania or excessive excitement. His work was reported in the *Medical Journal of Australia* and attracted little notice. But Danish, French and Italian psychiatrists became interested finally, and reported similar success.

Two British researchers discovered that sodium and potassium balances are disordered in depressed individuals. Cell sodium levels in depressives are found to be 50 per cent higher than normal. Manic patients had sodium levels three times over normal. Potassium levels were lower than they should have been. Giving these patients lithium, the scientists found that sodium levels decreased.

"Lithium is a simple, naturally occurring chemical, the third element and one of the groups of alkaline metals (such as sodium and potassium) on the periodic table," says an article, "Lithium vs. Mental Illness," in *The New York Times Magazine* for January 12, 1969. Edwin Diamond goes on to tell us that this mineral is the lightest known metal. It is found in rock formations and sea water. Potters use it as a glaze and it has other industrial uses as well.

During a routine survey in Texas as part of the federal government's report on nutrition early in 1969, scientists took urine specimens from many Texans, as well as taking samples of drinking water. The scientists decided they might as well check the drinking water samples for trace mineral content. And they found, according to *Medical World News* for October 15, 1971, that in the wet regions of the state there was almost no lithium in the drinking water. Moving into drier areas, they found increasing amounts of the trace metal.

The researchers knew that lithium can calm the "manic" or excited stage of manic-depressive illness. So they decided to check on mental hospital admissions in these areas. What they found astonished them. In the wet areas of Texas, where the average amount of lithium in the water was only 6 micrograms per liter, the rate of mental hospital admissions was 34.6 per 100,000. Moving into the drier areas, the average amount of lithium in drinking water rose to 60 micrograms per liter and the rate of mental hospital admissions fell to 24.9. In parts of the state where the lithium content of the water was as high as 160 micrograms per liter, mental hospital admissions fell to a surprising 16.3 per 100,000.

Going further in their search, the scientists tested the urine samples they had taken. Sure enough, as the amount of lithium in urine samples increased, the number of mental hospital admissions decreased. In the three counties with the highest lithium excretion, the lowest mental hospital admission figures prevailed. Earl Dawson, a Texas biochemist, reported these findings at a meeting of the American Medical Association in 1971. He was challenged by a specialist from the National Institutes of Mental Health who claimed that lithium is known to benefit only depressed patients while it may make schizophrenics worse. To us, this doesn't seem to negate Dr. Dawson's findings. Fewer mental patients probably means better mental health, no matter what particular form of mental illness the patients are suffering from.

Lithium was reported as useful in the treatment of alcoholism, according to *The New York Times* for June 22, 1973. Dr. Nathan S. Kline of Rockland State Hospital believes that it is often depression which causes alcoholism. Treating the patient with lithium may relieve the depression and make escape through alcohol unnecessary.

Dr. Kline has used the trace mineral extensively. He conducted a test in a Maine veterans hospital where 73 out-patients were treated with lithium in tablet form. These men had severe periodic drinking problems. Another similar group was given a tablet that looked like the mineral tablet but contained nothing of consequence. Some of the patients were studied for one year, some for two years.

"On the average," says the *Times*, "those who had been taking lithium had significantly fewer bouts of severe drinking than the others, Dr. Kline told a session of the 3rd annual conference of the National Institute of Alcohol Abuse and Alcoholism." It wasn't that the patients on lithium became teetotalers, but they had fewer drinking bouts severe enough to require hospitalization. About 73 per cent of those who got the "nothing" pill had at least one disabling drinking bout, while only 43 per cent of those who got the lithium had a similar bout. And those who were getting the lithium had significantly fewer such bouts than they had gone through in the previous year. There is no doubt, Dr. Kline said, that drinking problems decreased in the patients who were getting lithium, although none of the patients knew which group was taking this "drug" as the doctors call it.

The *Times* magazine article quotes a West Coast psychiatrist as saying, "We don't know if the mental state causes the chemical imbalance or if the chemical imbalance causes the mental state or if both are caused by something else. But once we find a drug that creates the right thymoleptic effect—that is, acts as a mood normalizer—then our traditional means of treatment will be outdated."

Lithium appears to be most effective for treating the manic stage of the manic-depressive illness. And, if given over long periods, it seems to decrease the number of depressive incidents and their severity. By now many thousands of people, the world around, are being treated with this simple, natural earth-mineral. In cases where there is danger of overdosage, urine and blood are monitored. In other cases, patients are apparently able to judge for themselves how to regulate their dosages. Like other minerals, hormones and vitamins, lithium appears to be a substance that must be taken for the rest of one's life if one is subject to depressive illness. It's not just a "treatment" which will "cure."

Considering all the work that has been done up to now on mental illness of various kinds and its relation to nutritional health and vitamin and mineral status, one cannot help but feel that lithium treatment is another step on the way to solving these widespread, extremely difficult health problems. Doesn't it seem possible that we will eventually be able to detect in individuals the tendency to need more than average amounts of certain vitamins and/or minerals, so that they can be supplied as needed in order to balance and set straight those workings of the body machinery that have gone awry? The Texas tests seemed to show that lithium taken every day in drinking water helps maintain such a balance. According to Karl Schütte, M.Sc., Ph.D., in *The Biology of Trace Minerals,* lithium occurs in extremely small amounts (from 0.01 to 10 ppm) in plants.

Dr. Fieve, in the above-named *Times* magazine article (November 25, 1973), although enthusiastic about lithium as a treatment for depression, did have this warning. "If people are going to rush in and use it inappropriately . . . there might be tragic results. I've had people call me and say, 'My brother's depressed—where can I get some lithium?' I tell them it should only be given after proper diagnosis and then it has to be closely monitored by an experienced M.D."

Medical Tribune for January 9, 1974 reports on a worldwide symposium on mental health in Geneva, Switzerland, at which a number of physicians and psychiatrists told of their experiences with lithium. Dr. Mogens Schou of Aarhus University, Copenhagen, Denmark, says that he "practices psychiatry by air mail" using lithium.

"The cost of keeping a patient on lithium for a year is about the same as a three-day stay in a hospital," he said. "So it offers an excellent cost-benefit ratio in reducing the morbidity associated with the affective disorders (mania and depression). But although lithium itself is cheap to use," the doctor went on, "there remains the problem of monitoring plasma (blood) concentration regularly, and the equipment and staff for this is not always available. We get around the difficulty by operating an air mail testing service."

Dr. Schou gives his patients a plastic tube taped to an

air mail letter. Periodically the patients send blood samples to a central point, where they are tested for too much or too little lithium in the blood. He is working with doctors as far away as Peru and Turkey. The blood sample reaches him in two or three days, and a warning is cabled back if the lithium level is found to be above or below what it should be.

The problem with lithium, as we have already found out, is that too much of it in the blood disturbs the balance between body fluids and certain other minerals, including potassium and sodium. The body has very delicate mechanisms for regulating this balance and any disruption can cause serious trouble—nausea, vomiting, for example. Even with these symptoms, says Dr. Schou, one can go on treating the patient with lithium if enough attention is given to levels of the trace mineral in the blood. It must be carefully watched.

In patients who may have tremors, they might find it embarrassing in public with hands unable to hold a coffee cup without shaking. So Dr. Schou gives the larger dose of lithium before bedtime and a smaller dose in the morning. Sometimes the patient is thirsty or urinates excessively. There seems to be no kidney complication involved, reports Dr. Schou.

Another symptom may be swelling of the thyroid gland or goiter—another indication that body mechanisms are being disrupted. Dr. Schou gives his patients thyroxine for the goiter. Weight gain seems to be another problem. We presume this means that the lithium causes water to accumulate in the body, but we do not know for sure. In any case, with very careful management and frequent testing, Dr. Schou is apparently having success in his treatment of depression with lithium.

Another Danish physician, Prof. Ole Rafaelsen of Copenhagen, reported on three seemingly unrelated conditions which also are benefitted by lithium: Ménière's disease, Huntington's Chorea and a condition called *tardive dyskinesia,* which is a disease involving involuntary movements. In treating this condition, the amino acid tryptophane is used along with the lithium.

No one knows why the lithium treatment benefits victims of Ménière's Syndrome. This is a disorder of the inner ear, involving deafness, vertigo and tinnitus or ringing in the ears. It was first described in 1861 by Prosper Ménière. Sometimes the victim also suffers from nausea, vomiting and nystagmus, which is an uncontrollable rolling of the eyeballs. It is believed that Ménière's disease may be caused by a disturbance of water balance and those minerals which control this mechanism—chiefly sodium and potassium.

Dr. Rafaelsen conducted a test of 40 patients with Ménière's disease. He gave them a form of lithium. Ten of them gave up almost at once, suffering from side effects. Twenty-one remained on the lithium therapy with beneficial results. Nine discontinued the treatment after an average of four months since they could see no benefits.

Of the 21 successful treatments, 16 of these patients are still taking lithium, the treatment period ranging from 3 to 30 months. Five have been able to stop all treatment after 10 to 18 months with total disappearance of symptoms. Dr. Rafaelsen says that one patient has gained 30 pounds, but the 52-year-old woman, who had suffered from Ménière's disease for eight years, insists on continuing the lithium because of the relief it has brought her. In most cases where patients gain weight, states Dr. Rafaelsen, it is not more than 10 to 20 pounds.

Dr. Rafaelsen reminded the physicians in his audience that his experiments are preliminary. He has not done any "controlled experiments" in which some patients are given the drug and the results are compared with a group of patients who get a pill with nothing in it. But he says that his trial with 40 patients could hardly have produced such results if the patients were responding psychologically just to the effect of "something new" in the way of treatment.

Patients with Huntington's Chorea have shown improvement, according to tests by Dr. Per Dalen of St. Jorgen's Hospital, Hisings Becka, Sweden. Thirty patients were treated with lithium and 60 per cent showed improvement. Huntington's Chorea is a nervous disorder, supposedly inherited, which usually appears late in life. It involves irregular, involuntary movements along with disturbed speech and brain function.

"It is said that of the 1,000 or more people in America affected with Huntington's Chorea, all descended from three men, probably brothers, who came to America in about 1630," states *The Book of Health*. "The descendants of this trio scattered over the New England states, and many were involved in early witchcraft trials, because the odd symptoms of the disease aroused the suspicions of superstitious persons."

Let us reiterate that we do not know of any source of lithium with which laymen can treat themselves. This mineral should be administered by a doctor. If you suspect that you may be suffering from manic depression, by all means ask your physician about lithium. If he is unfamiliar with its use, show him this book.

The fact that you may be depressed does not necessarily mean that you are suffering from manic depression. Lots of things can cause less serious depression and there is much you can do on your own to conquer it. Maybe you're just bored. If so, get out and do something worthwhile (volunteer to work for the Red Cross, to read to the sick in a local hospital, etc.), meet people, get involved in some worthwhile or engrossing activity which will take your mind off your own troubles! You will find there are many people in worse shape than you are in.

Maybe you're not eating properly or not getting enough exercise. Check your diet. Did you eat a good, nourishing, high-protein breakfast, lunch and dinner?

Or did you just load up on sugar? Have you eliminated from your meals all those high-carbohydrate traps that bring about low blood sugar—one of the commonest reasons for depression? How much coffee do you drink? Are your snacks the good, nourishing ones like cheese, nuts, seeds, fresh fruits and vegetables? Do you get enough sleep? Are you doing work that interests you and stimulates you? Do you have some family problem that fills you with resentment every day? Is the local noise and air pollution getting you down?

There are many reasons for transient depression. Give yourself a good chance to lick any of these problems before you go to your physician and demand lithium. There is a lot that you can do before you go looking for a "magic pill."

CHAPTER 20

Fluoride

IN 1939, a monumental book appeared entitled *Nutrition and Physical Degeneration*. It was written by a dentist, Weston Price, who traveled around the world to study the effect of diet on the health of human teeth. He visited Peruvian Indians and American Indians on our West coast. He studied the Pacific Islanders, including Polynesians, Melanesians, Australian Aborigines and New Zealand Maori. He went to isolated spots in Switzerland, whose inhabitants had almost no contact with the outside world, and islands off the coast of Ireland, where diet and the way of life had not changed in many generations.

Dr. Price examined Africans living as their ancestors have lived for thousands of years, comparing them with Africans who now live in cities and eat a "civilized" diet. He studied the Eskimos. Throughout the years of his travels, he took photographs which appear on 135 pages of this 500-page book.

And Dr. Price's findings—amply confirmed by his photographs—prove unequivocally that tooth decay is the product of modern refined and processed carbohydrates and all the foods made from them—white sugar and white flour chiefly, along with processed cereals. It doesn't matter much what the primitive people were eating—mostly vegetarian or mostly carnivorous diets—or mixtures of the two; as long as processed carbohydrates had no part in the diet, tooth decay as such was

196

almost unknown. As soon as "white man's food" or "store-bought food" was introduced into the diets of these incredibly sturdy, well-developed and healthy people, tooth decay followed with agonizing results.

In the next generation it's not just teeth but bone structure as well which degenerates, resulting in air passages not wide enough for breathing, mouths too narrow for a full set of teeth, pinched nostrils, long, pinched faces rather than round, full ones. "Physical degeneration" is what Dr. Price calls this. Although he was not a physician, he found abundant evidence that processed foods also brought other ill-health in many forms—chiefly TB—which affected many of the people he studied. He found that native Africans lose their immunity to epidemic African diseases when the second generation on refined foods comes along.

Not once does the word "fluoride" appear in Dr. Price's massive book. He was apparently unaware of the possible effect of fluoride in food and water as relating to tooth decay, so he took no notice of the level of this trace element in the diet and water of the people he studied. So there is no chance that fluoride or lack of fluoride in their diets and water supply could have influenced the evidence he brought back.

Since Dr. Price's time, thousands of studies have been made and duly reported in medical and scientific literature, which confirm his research and show that human beings are no more susceptible to tooth decay than are wild animals, so long as their diets contain only the same natural foods which wild animals eat, with the exception that humans cook some of theirs. So well known is the ability of sticky, refined sweets and starches to create holes in teeth that something called a "cariogenic diet" is routinely used in laboratories the world over to induce tooth decay in animals. This is the same kind of diet many of us eat every day. Our children especially are prone to eat relatively enormous amounts of refined sweets and starches with disastrous effects on teeth.

Quite recently a great deal of research is turning up the facts about other diseases than tooth decay which are caused directly by the ingestion of huge amounts of refined carbohydrates, rather than the natural starches and sweets which animals and primitive peoples eat: roots, nuts, seeds, berries and fruits. A group of British physicians have presented convincing evidence that many diseases other than tooth decay follow the introduction of refined carbohydrate foods as regularly as day follows night.

Twenty years after an individual has left his native culture and ways of eating, and has succumbed to the lure of inexpensive, easily obtained refined carbohydrate foods, he achieves rapidly the degenerative status of industrialized man where digestive diseases and circulatory diseases are concerned. He may get peptic ulcer, diverticular disease, colitis, constipation, heart and circulatory conditions, etc., all of which are almost completely unknown to primitive people living on wholly natural diets.

American biologists are as conversant as those of other countries with the facts presented above, so far as tooth decay is concerned. *American scientists know what causes tooth decay.* Dentists warn their patients that sugar and sticky starches are not good for teeth. But it has seldom occurred to most of them that food substances which cause such terrible destruction of teeth and bone structure could also be responsible for the other diseases listed above. Most dentists and physicians, alas, have little knowledge about nutrition and seem to care little about its effects on human health.

In the late 1930's, when a Mellon Institute research fellow discovered that people with fluoride in their water supply had fewer cavities than those without fluoride, the entire public health establishment jumped on the bandwagon and eventually endorsed general, nationwide fluoridation of water supplies as *the only effective method of preventing tooth decay!* By 1950, the American Dental Association and a number of professional societies had "endorsed" water fluoridation.

Meanwhile, industries which make most of their profits from refined and processed carbohydrates were understandably pleased that fluoridation of all drinking water could solve the nation's problem of tooth decay and would, at the same time, allow their profits to sky-rocket. Children could saturate themselves in soft drinks, candy and desserts because the fluoride in the drinking water would control their tooth decay. Well, almost control it. For some of the evidence that soon began to appear challenged the basic assumption that doing nothing but fluoridating water would end such-and-such a percentage of tooth decay.

It was well known at the time fluoridation was introduced that getting too much fluoride would cause poisoning. The first symptom is tooth mottling (a common sight in the Texas Panhandle, where water is high in fluoride naturally)—an unsightly defect in teeth which cannot be eliminated. Yet, in spite of this, we were told that dumping sodium fluoride in a city or town water supply—at the waterworks—would guarantee that everyone in the community—young and old, sick and well—would get "exactly" the right amount of fluoride, whether they drank one glass or dozens of glasses of water each day. In vain did anti-fluoridationists point out that the amount of fluoride any individual gets depends on the amount of water he drinks and the amount of fluoride in that glass of water. Anyone who drinks milk, fruit juice, soft drinks or booze instead of water will not get any fluoride from his city drinking water. And the individual who, for one reason or another, drinks enormous amounts of water is almost bound to get too much fluoride.

Public health officials continue to insist that "the

average American" drinks a certain amount of water, therefore, everybody in a city whose water supply contains 1.5 ppm of fluoride is bound to get the same amount of fluoride—and that is bound to be the "right" amount to protect children from tooth decay up to the age of 18 or thereabouts.

In vain did the anti-fluoridationists point out that it was very unlikely that water works could so manipulate their machinery that exactly the same amount of fluoride would be present in everybody's drinking water as it came from the faucet. Pro-fluoridationists said the level of fluoride in the water *could and would be maintained at exactly the same level year after year.*

Early in the fluoridation game its proponents warned against getting too much fluoride. Getting a bit too much brings the tooth mottling that we mentioned. And this is likely to appear in a considerable number of all children getting water fluoridated at 1.5 ppm.

In an article in the June 1968 issue of the *American Journal of Clinical Nutrition,* four researchers did a careful survey of the food eaten by 2,655 people in a Puerto Rican slum. They assessed the amount of protein, fat, calories, vitamins and minerals these people were getting at mealtime, then, by means of medical examinations, they discovered what each person's health picture was. Among their findings was that "Dental caries (decayed teeth) were common and increasingly frequent with age. Over 40 years of age, a decreasing prevalence of caries was observed. This was due to the increasing number of missing teeth. Pregnant and lactating women showed the highest prevalence of tooth decay." An accompanying table showed that 2.9 per cent of all the 2,655 people were suffering from tooth mottling. In the 10- to 14-year-old group, 11 per cent of all the children showed this symptom of too much fluoride.

Since there was nothing in the article to indicate where the fluoride poisoning was coming from, we wrote to a professor at the University of Puerto Rico for an explanation. He informed us that the water in that area of Puerto Rico had been fluoridated for 15 years. At first, he said, they used 1 ppm of fluoride, the amount recommended for use in the U.S. But then they decided that the hot climate would probably make most people drink more water than they would in a cooler climate, so they reduced the fluoride to 0.7 to 0.8 ppm.

"However," he continued, "there is evidence, although not particularly from the area studied, that the concentration of fluoride in the water varies from none to 2 to 3 ppm *due to irregularities in the fluoridation process.*" (Italics ours).

According to *The New York Times*, September 27, 1972, the president of the American Dental Association has discovered that many of the nation's supposedly fluoridated water supplies "might not be fluoridated" after all. "Children in these communities are growing up with far more decayed teeth than expected," he said, referring to surveys made in six states. "Many communities that were supposedly fluoridating were not doing so at all or only sporadically. . . . What was found in these six states has application in every state in the nation."

He goes on to say that it's possible nobody has ordered the waterworks people not to put fluoride in the water. But, instead, maybe the waterworks personnel are just not highly trained enough to make certain that all the water contains just the right amount of fluoride all the time. In other words, even if there is no malfunction in the machinery, the people operating the machinery may not know what they are doing, so you could easily not get very much fluoride—or you might get too much! Can you think of a better testimonial for recommending bottled water?

"A high intake of fluoride is known to cause severe skeletal fluorosis," says Dr. H. A. Cook in the October 9, 1971 issue of *Lancet*, "but the actual fluoride intake required to produce fluorosis is unknown. I have shown that tea-drinking in Britain causes a high fluoride intake in both children and adults, maximum intakes in children surveyed reaching nearly 6 mg. daily in unfluoridated areas and nearly 7 mg. daily in fluoridated areas. It is possible that fluoride intake from tea may be sufficient to cause fluorosis, and I report here a case which gives some evidence of this."

Dr. Cook describes the case of a 55-year-old woman who had been crippled by arthritis for 25 years. Twelve years ago she moved to an area with more fluoride in the water, since she had been told that fluoride is good for teeth and bones. The water there contained 0.67 ppm or just about half the 1.5 ppm recommended in the U.S. The lady drank from 3 to 4 pints of tea daily, which would be roughly 6 to 8 cups.

Tests of her excretion of fluorine showed that she was excreting 1.5 to 2 ppm of fluoride, which, according to authorities quoted by Dr. Cook, indicates that fluoride is being retained—that is, bones and teeth are taking it up and using it. She stopped drinking tea. Within three months she told Dr. Cook that her arthritic pain had diminished to the point where she was almost able to do without drugs entirely. She was now able to move about so well that she took a job involving lots of walking. Within six months she was virtually free from pain and doing without drugs almost entirely. One year after she stopped drinking tea, there was no further improvement, but there had been no deterioration, and she was able to do without drugs entirely, except in emergencies.

"Possibly," says Dr. Cook, "some cases of pain diagnosed as rheumatism or arthritis may be due to subclinical fluorosis which is not radiologically demonstrated (that is, cannot be seen on X-rays)."

The Journal of the American Medical Association (November 13, 1972) reported on two cases of grievous harm apparently wrought on people with kidney disorders who drank excessive amounts of water which was fluoridated. The authors, Dr. Luis I. Juncos and Dr. James V. Donacio, Jr., physicians at the Mayo Clinic in Minnesota, wrote: "It is generally agreed that water fluoridation is safe for persons with normal kidneys. Systemic fluorosis (poisoning by fluoride) in patients with diminished renal function, however, seems a reasonable possibility. In such patients, fluoride may be retained with resulting higher tissue fluoride levels than in persons with normal renal (kidney) function, especially in patients with renal insufficiency who live in areas of the world that have augmented fluoride content in the available water."

They describe an 18-year-old boy and a 17-year-old girl, both suffering from mottled teeth. The condition of the bones of both patients was suggestive of more advanced fluoride poisoning. Say the authors, "The question is whether the chronic excess fluoride intake caused the renal damage (either directly or indirectly) or whether the systemic fluorosis was due to impaired renal function."

The boy habitually drank about two gallons of water daily from an artesian well. He suffered from perennial thirst and excessive urination. The water in the well contained 2.6 ppm of fluoride. A dental expert who examined his teeth pronounced them free from decay, but he found some loss of bone structure in the jaw and possibly loss of tooth socket cortex. The boy was told to stop drinking so much water and to drink only fluoride-free water. A year later he was drinking only about one gallon a day and his symptoms had subsided.

The girl had more serious problems. Since infancy she had always drunk large amounts of water and had suffered from recurrent urinary tract infections. The fluoride of her drinking water was 1.7 ppm. She had protein in her urine and an excess of nitrogenous compounds in her blood. Her doctors operated on her ureter, the tube conveying urine from the kidneys to the bladder. A year later she was in serious condition, eating a low protein diet but still drinking enormous amounts of water.

The Mayo Clinic doctors said of their patients, "It is postulated that the renal insufficiency which resulted in the large intake of fluoride-containing water and reduced excretion of fluoride combined to produce systemic fluorosis." Thus, it is apparent that many people who drink large amounts of water—untreated diabetics for example—may be suffering from a variety of ills which no doctor can diagnose without knowing the fluoride content of the water supply, and then knowing whether or not the fluoride is causing the damage. If you are in such a predicament, you can switch over to unfluoridated water and see if the symptoms disappear. If they do, then it's rather obvious that it's the fluoride in the water which is producing them.

It was, of course, inevitable that someone would suggest putting fluoride in toothpaste. Pro-fluoridationists thought this was a grand idea, but anti-fluoridationists warned that fluoridated toothpaste should not be sold in localities where water was fluoridated. But no one paid any attention to this warning, and fluoridated toothpastes became the vogue, no matter whether there was fluoride in the water supply or not. Then vitamin pills began to feature fluoride. And chewing gum. Then, of course, there were the countless products in the supermarket packed in water that was fluoridated. And, of course, more fluoride from air pollution. Some foods, like tea, already contain considerable fluoride. Thus, when you consider all of these sources, how can anyone tell how many children are actually getting "the right" amount of fluoride?

In the September 25, 1971 issue of *Lancet*, Dr. T. K. Day and Dr. P. Powell-Jackson point out that using fluoride toothpaste may result in children consuming as much as 2.4 to 2.6 mg. of fluoride daily from the toothpaste. In areas where water is fluoridated with 1 ppm ot fluoride, children are already getting 2.2 to 3.2 mg. of fluoride. Adding the fluoride from toothpaste to the fluoride in drinking water might easily result in an intake considerably higher than that which is considered safe, the physicians state. They point out that a daily intake of more than 2 mg. of fluoride during childhood leads to tooth mottling; taking up to 4 mg. daily for five to 10 years produces osteosclerosis (a diseased condition in which the bone becomes hard and heavy). And taking more than 20 mg. of fluoride daily during adolescence results in crippling fluorosis, they added. They also stated that they have found evidence that very low levels of fluoride produce goiters. In villages where goiter was common and everyone was getting about the same amount of iodine, they studied the amount of fluoride in the water supply and found there was considerably more goiter in places where the water contained fluoride —even at very low levels—never greater than 0.4 ppm.

"Perhaps in our enthusiasm for preventive dentistry, we have forgotten that the level of fluoride intake which is effective in preventing (tooth decay) is dangerously close to the level which produces harmful effects," the British scientists say.

Six children and one adult, all suffering from allergic reactions, were relieved of their symptoms when they eliminated the source of fluoride, which, in these cases, was toothpaste and vitamin preparations containing fluoride, according to an article in *Annals of Allergy* (July 1967). The authors—Dr. J. J. Shea, Dr. S. M. Gillespie and Dr. G. L. Waldbott—tell us that two earlier researchers reported allergies in 1 per cent of 672 pregnant women to whom they gave fluoride tablets to prevent dental decay. Dr. Waldbott, a leading allergist, has reported in the past on patients of his whose skin rashes were due to fluoridated drinking water. Another doctor is quoted as having found allergy in one patient out of 20 to whom he was giving fluoride.

Still another allergist found that 133 of his patients were allergic to the fluoride in their toothpaste. With 32 of these, he eliminated the allergy by discontinuing the toothpaste, then brought it on again by telling them to use the toothpaste again. He did this six times. Each time the allergy returned when the toothpaste was used; it disappeared when it was not used.

In the *Annals* article, we are told of a 48-year-old man who regularly got hives every morning shortly after breakfast. He had been using a toothpaste that contained fluoride. He discontinued it and within six days was completely free of the allergy. Three years later, he inadvertently used the fluoride toothpaste and the hives came back. He was persuaded to agree to a test of his sensitivity to fluoride. A local pharmacist prepared three unmarked bottles containing distilled water and the patient was told to take, every day, one tablespoon from the first bottle one week, the second bottle the second week, the third bottle the third week. He did, with no reactions except from Bottle No. 2, which gave him hives immediately. They disappeared at the end of the week when he began to use Bottle No. 3. Bottle No. 2 contained added fluoride.

The other patients discussed in the article were children who were either using fluoridated toothpaste or taking vitamin drops containing fluoride. These are the kind prescribed by doctors. The symptoms included rashes, persistent bloody diarrhea, ulcers in the mouth, swelling of the salivary glands, cramps, headaches, etc. When the toothpaste or the drops were discontinued, the symptoms disappeared in every case. One girl got her symptoms back the day she used a fluoride toothpaste by mistake.

The authors pinpoint another disturbing result of taking fluorides in toothpaste, pills or drinking water. When inorganic fluorides combine with the hydrochloric acid in the stomach, hydrofluoric acid is formed. This is a very irritating and corrosive substance which can damage the lining of the stomach and the upper digestive tract. People who tend to have too much hydrochloric acid in their stomachs would, of course, be the first to suffer from such a symptom.

As we have stated, no one knows how much fluoride any individual is getting in his food. Recently, the FDA has asked that labels on food cans must contain information on exactly what is inside the can in the way of protein, fats, carbohydrates, vitamins and minerals which are officially essential. No mention of fluorides. So you still will not be able to tell how much fluoride you are getting.

Recently, a University of Montana scientist tested the amounts of fluoride in pet food. He found the levels varied from 11 ppm in Alpo Chopped Beef to 193 ppm in Ken-L-Ration stew dog food. And 25 ppm in 9-Lives Tuna and up to 83 ppm in Puss n' Boots. Testing the bones of pet animals for fluoride, he found the range of values to be from 84 ppm to 1,535 ppm for dogs, and 74 ppm to 1,190 ppm for cats. There was a tendency for the amount of fluoride to increase with age. Concerned veterinarians began to wonder whether these high levels of fluoride might have anything to do with bone, kidney and other ailments in pets. Has the fluoride content of human food gone up as it has in the pet food? How can we know? Nor do we know why the fluoride content of some of these foods was so high. Nor do we know whether the dogs and cats in question were also drinking fluoridated water. Some of the pets might even be getting vitamin pills containing fluoride.

Thirty-two cases of early pre-skeletal fluorosis due to pollution from nearby fertilizer factories and an iron foundry were reported by Dr. George Waldbott of Harper Hospital, Detroit, at the 2nd International Clean

Air Congress of the International Union of Air Pollution Prevention Association. Excessive exposure to fluoride was established by high fluoride levels in food, fly ash and water, and by visible damage to crops, livestock and materials. All of the 32 patients had identical symptoms. There was a gradual progressive feeling of general ill health and exhaustion, which ended in complete disability. Nearly all patients reported pain and stiffness in the spine, with restriction of spinal movements and arthritis in other joints. They also had numbness and tingling sensations in arms, legs and shoulders. The muscular power of hands and legs was impaired.

Migraine-like headaches on both sides were the complaint of 20 of the 32 patients, as well as visual disturbances not improved by glasses. Eighteen had digestive tract symptoms, diagnosed by their physicians as gallbladder disease, intestinal flu or a stricture of the bowel. Several of them could trace their symptoms from a time when they ate food contaminated by fluoride from the nearby factories.

Laboratory tests showed almost nothing, as they do in cases of early chronic fluorosis. But biopsy material showed a high fluoride content of bone and soft tissues. In one case the amount of fluoride being excreted in the urine dropped from an average of 19.9 mg. to an average of 2.6 mg. when the patient moved away from the polluted area.

Dr. Waldbott, as quoted in *Medical Tribune*, April 21, 1971, says that chronic poisoning from airborne pollutants is generally difficult to attribute to its cause, because it develops slowly and insidiously with vague symptoms that mimic numerous other diseases, often without specific clinical and laboratory features.

In an earlier article in *GP*, a medical journal, Dr. Waldbott states that, during the past 30 years, fluoride has increased as a pollutant in water and air and that it is a familiar ingredient in many new drugs. Practically every food contains fluoride, he says, and some—like tea and seafood—contain up to 100 ppm of fluoride.

On May 12, 1965 at Hotel Biltmore, New York City, and reported in that day's edition of the *New York Journal-American,* the Medical-Dental Committee of the Greater New York Committee Opposed to Fluoridation demonstrated a new lab technique which enables scientists to record what happens to cell tissue when it comes in contact with fluoride. The study was accomplished through the use of time-lapse cinephotomicrography. Dr. Jonathan Forman, editor of *Clinical Physiology* and a former president of the American College of Allergists, acted as moderator at the showing. He discussed this Time-Lapse Research Foundation study in greater detail in the March-April, 1965 issue of *National Fluoridation News.*

"What one sees on the film, at first," said the newspaper, "are living cells growing in a normal fashion. Then fluoride is added. It then becomes clear that a 'stress' of some sort has been introduced and that the living tissue is actively responding in an effort to overcome the stress.

"What has happened, according to Dr. Jonathan Forman, is that the fluorine ions have entered the 'distressed' cells and blocked various vital enzymes, thus breaking the chain of enzyme reactions which control all life processes.

"Some cells die immediately," the newspaper continues. "In others, the metabolic activity slows down and finally ends. Every cell, according to Dr. Forman, is either killed or has its normal growth altered."

In the April, 1972 issue of *American Forests,* Dale Burk writes about what happened to a corner of Montana where an aluminum company had been pouring fluorine into the air at the rate of 2,500 pounds a day for some 15 years. Infrared photographs showed extensive damage to thousands of acres of forestland, some of it in national parks. Food grown in the area showed accumulations of as much as 226 ppm of fluoride. Deer from the dying forests have been examined and found to be suffering from "serious deterioration of their teeth and bones because of the fluorides." Forest service officials, who first noticed the damage in 1957, did nothing about it until 1969. In addition to the damage to flora and fauna there was, of course, incalculable damage to human beings during this time.

Dr. Underwood tells us in *Trace Elements in Human and Animal Nutrition* that fluoride is used in the manufacture of steel, paper, textiles and plastics. Burning any of these might well increase the fluoride in air pollution, which would eventually end up in water, as all persistent pollutants do. So in any area where solid waste is burned in incinerators, one should expect that fluoride will increasingly pollute air and drinking water.

Those who oppose fluoridation point out that, in waters where fluoride appears naturally, it appears in conjunction with calcium and magnesium, which are the natural components of such "hard" waters. To use sodium fluoride in water which contains little calcium and magnesium is taking a chance, since we have little knowledge as to the synergistic effect of these various minerals. We have been told that calcium appears to be a guarantee against harm from fluoride. Therefore, say the opponents of fluoridation, to dump fluoride into a water with no regard for other minerals present is courting disaster. Nonsense, say the proponents, the fluoride ion is the fluoride ion. They insist that fluoride dumped into city water will guarantee comparative freedom from tooth decay, at least in pre-teen children. But there has always been considerable confusion as to how long the immunity lasts, with many statisticians pointing out that fluoridation only postpones tooth decay and that, after several years, the 16-year-olds will probably have as much decay as the 18-year-olds.

And so the battle rages, almost destroying whole city governments in some areas as they debate whether or not to fluoridate the city water. Proponents call opponents faddists and cranks, regardless of their academic and scientific credentials. Opponents claim that drinking water is for the purpose of slaking thirst and may not legally be used to administer drugs.

Lost in the controversy is the question of the possible role of fluoride in the weird witches brew of pollutants present in most urban air and water. There are millions of them. And no one has any idea what combinations of one or two or more may presage in the way of danger. We have presented throughout this book much evidence of a network of relationships prevailing among trace minerals. You get a bit too much of one and it throws out the balance of two others. You get a bit too little of something else and you face the threat of harm from something quite different which may then be present in too large a concentration.

In the light of all this, it seems the height of folly to dump into the only drinking water available, deliberately and with a promise of vast health benefits, a poison whose relationship with the millions of other environmental poisons has not even begun to be investigated, if indeed it can ever be sorted out.

And it seems to be an incredible public health bungle to advocate such a measure in order to reduce incidence of a non-fatal and non-infectious disease, whose cause is well known to science and dentistry. It's a disease which could be stopped in its tracks by simply returning, generally speaking, to the kinds of diets our ancestors ate ages before refined carbohydrates appeared on the scene. Fortunately, there is a nationwide movement afoot to do just this. And it's gaining headway every year.

On November 2, 1970, Ralph Nader, the outspoken consumer advocate, spoke on the environmental crisis in Sioux Falls, South Dakota. "The U.S. Public Health

Service has a totally paranoic mind on (the subject of fluoridation)," he said. "And it's very serious, because if it's paranoid on this issue, what is it going to be on other issues? . . . all those who are for fluoridation think that those who are against fluoridation are kooks, psychotics. . . . Now in *Science* magazine about two years ago there was a report that the U.S. Public Health Service had a file on all the major critics of fluoridation with all kinds of extraneous personal information which it then released strategically to various sources and media throughout the country. The Public Health Service, unfortunately, has locked itself into a position where it has made this statement on the record that there is absolutely no hazard to fluoridating public water supplies and the matter is closed. Now that, of course, is immediately an anti-scientific or unscientific approach. The matter must never be closed. . . .

"One of my legal associates once made a study of how the fluoridation issue is decided," Nader continued. "It was printed in the *George Washington Law Review* (showing that fluoridation) was decided basically by a particularly acute lobbying effort by a number of dentists who stampeded the Public Health Service into the decision. Once the Public Health Service had gone on record, it could never be proved wrong. It would lose too much face. If the Public Health Service was proved wrong, what would people think about the Public Health Service in all the other things they are doing? It's a very pathetic situation, unfortunately. . . .

"I've been told by a number of scientists—some of them Nobel laureates—that they have grave doubts that this is the most effective way to combat dental caries in children, that there are much more efficient, much more comprehensive ways, without exposing the whole population. . . . Perhaps the crux of the argument is the following: that there are better ways to cut down the dental caries in the subject population without exposing

80 per cent of the population to it. One of the principles of ecology is you do not intrude new elements into an ecological pattern unless you have an awfully good reason to and unless the benefits far outweigh the costs. . . .

"I've often wondered," he said, "why all the people who are for fluoridation never say anything about soft drinks, never say anything about bleached white flour, never say anything about manipulations which are leading to the production of so many dental caries in our children. That's something I think should be severely emphasized because it's not only the production of diets, it's the malnutrition of even well-to-do children around the country."

Is fluorine/fluoride necessary in human nutrition? Well, as we have indicated, it may curtail or postpone tooth decay in some children. However, if these children eat sticky, gooey sweets all day long, no amount of fluoride is going to keep them from making frequent trips to the dentist.

CHAPTER 21

Beryllium

ACCORDING TO Dr. Henry A. Schroeder, as reported in *Science News*, July 21, 1973, beryllium is the most highly toxic substance with which he has worked. Beryllium gets into lungs and causes inflammation; it has been known to cause cancer. People who are regularly exposed to beryllium are workers in the beryllium and coal industries and those breathing exhausts from rocket fuels at Cape Canaveral. It is also used in ceramics, copper alloys, computers, household appliances, ball-point pens. Apparently none of these items themselves are any cause for worry, but workers in plants where beryllium is processed are subject to a lung disease which can be fatal.

Medical World News, October 26, 1973, described a meeting of the Society for Occupational and Environmental Health, which was called to discuss beryllium contamination as an occupational hazard. All experts agree that the metal is toxic but no one knows why or at what levels it might be safe.

Yet, the Public Health Service reports that, in 1970, 30,000 of us were exposed to beryllium at work. The story is much the same as that of cadmium. The metal did not pose any threat to man until it began to be important for industry. Exposure to it became a threat because it was long-term exposure and in relatively enormous amounts, something which had never happened before in man's history on earth, so he has developed no protection against it. By the 1930's, cases of lung damage were reported in Europe. In 1946, cases of "delayed" beryllium poisoning were reported among makers of fluorescent lights where beryllium is used.

In acute poisonings the metal can produce skin ulcers, eye ulcers, severe lung pneumonitis, colds, laryngitis, pharyngitis and tracheobronchitis. All these are reversible if exposure is stopped. Chronic effects are: pneumonitis, cough, chest pain, general weakness, lung disorders, heart enlargement, congestive heart failure, enlargement of liver and spleen, cyanosis, clubbing of the fingers, kidney stones, along with other disabling effects.

A temporary official level of exposure was set in 1949 —2 micrograms of beryllium per cubic foot of air over an 8-hr. period. This is still the official level, although no one knows if this level is safe. It's generally accepted that even this level has never been met by industry. In fact, at a large beryllium plant in Pennsylvania, levels of beryllium in the air soar to thousands of times this level. The government agency responsible for monitoring such levels simply does not do its job. They have 4 million working places to monitor and only 1,000 men to perform the job, they say. Organized labor protests that the administration does not hit industry with fines or penalties when they find transgressions. And the administration says, well, yes, they generally rely on voluntary compliance with the rules.

Requests for records of victims of beryllium are refused. The disease is not recognized by physicians, so much of it may be wrongly diagnosed. Chronic beryllium poisoning may not develop until 25 years after exposure, so after he becomes seriously ill no one can really tell how much beryllium a victim has been exposed to or when.

The Beryllium Case Register lists 837 individuals, only six of them listed since 1966, so the official level of pollution may possibly be a safe one. Current research seems to show that exposure to beryllium may affect the immune reaction of some people, so that they become more susceptible to infections. Dr. Samuel Epstein of Case Western Reserve thinks such ideas are beside the point. He says, "Beryllium is very toxic and . . . exposure of all workers should be limited drastically. It is dangerous to think you can screen certain people out and leave others exposed."

There seem to be, as well, record numbers of cancer cases among beryllium workers: cancers of liver, bile duct and gallbladder and lung cancers.

In *Internal Medicine News,* February 15, 1972, a National Cancer Institute researcher reported the findings of cancer-causing substances in water supplies and a correlation between those levels and cancer figures in surrounding communities. Beryllium was correlated with bone cancer, breast and uterine cancer. Lead was correlated with kidney cancer, leukemias, lymphomas, stomach, intestinal and ovarian cancers. Cadmium was correlated most closely and frequently with cancer deaths. Nickel was correlated with oral cancer and intestinal cancer. Arsenic was correlated with larynx cancer, eye cancer and a kind of leukemia. Dr. John W. Berg, who made the report, reminds us that such figures are not absolute proof of cause and effect relationships.

The New York Times for October 29, 1972 tells the story of one Pennsylvania plant in which men are dying from beryllium poisoning. At Hazelton, the industry was welcomed because of widespread unemployment. The one doctor who foresaw health problems was ignored. Today he is convinced that a number of other workers have died of beryllium poisoning and that two former patients died of it, although he could not prove it. A *Times* story on March 18, 1973 describes a strike of the union workers at the plant, demanding protection from beryllium exposure. In 1971, readings of as much as

1,310 mcg., rather than the official level of 2 mcg. were made in some parts of the Hazelton building.

And another article in the *Times* (April 9, 1974) states: "One of the best-known occupational health hazards—beryllium—is being used in at least two fast-growing products that could expose unsuspecting workers and consumers to the metal's toxic fumes and dust." The two products are mantles for gas camping lanterns and dental alloys that substitute for gold in making inlays, bridges and crowns. Such products are generally not labeled as to their beryllium content and users are, therefore, not aware of the potential danger.

Kyle Griggs, a scientist at the University of California's Lawrence Livermore Laboratory, has found the camping lantern mantles release potentially hazardous amounts of beryllium fumes, the *Times* reports. The metal is used to harden the delicate, ashlike structure of the mantle. Griggs said that, when a new mantle is lit, most of the beryllium (about 400 mcg.) is released in the first 15 minutes. Since the lantern is usually in a confined space, such as a tent, it exposes the camper to fairly high levels of the metal, especially if he is near the light. Griggs suggests that a new mantle should be lit in an open area and left to burn for about five minutes before bringing the lantern inside.

Dental alloys containing beryllium are mainly a risk to dental laboratory technicians and dentists, especially if the alloy is ground and polished in a dental laboratory that lacks exhaust ventilation, the *Times* continues. But patients who require extensive dental work may be exposed to potentially harmful amounts of beryllium, since the alloys are often used instead of the higher-priced gold.

Dr. Joseph P. Moffa and his colleagues at the United States Public Health Service Hospital in San Francisco found that nine out of 10 alloys that were tested contained beryllium. This ranged from 1 per cent to nearly

217

2 per cent of the alloys' contents, the *Times* says. "Dr. Moffa's tests showed that a laboratory worker might be exposed to levels two and three times greater than the Federal standard, with levels in the breathing zone 60 to 160 times what the Atomic Energy Commission recommends," the *Times* reports.

Dr. Homayoun Kazemi, director of the U.S. Beryllium Case Registry at the Massachusetts General Hospital, said that "many of the 8,000 workplaces where beryllium is used are not abiding by the Federal exposure standard." He added that many of the beryllium disease cases are not correctly diagnosed because the symptoms resemble so many other conditions and because beryllium exposure is often not included in the patient's medical history. Dr. Kazemi said that failure to recognize beryllium disease was a virtual certainty in a case such as the dental alloys, where the workers are unaware of their beryllium exposure, the *Times* says.

On April 8, 1974, the Health Research Group, affiliated with Ralph Nader's consumer protection organization, asked the Food and Drug Administration for a report on the safety of dental alloys. They also requested that the contents of such alloys be disclosed on packages and in advertising, with proper labeling as to how to use the materials safely. And the American Dental Association's Council on Dental Materials and Devices is currently studying the new alloys.

Dr. G. L. Waldbott says in *Health Effects of Environmental Pollutants* that beryllium is used in roentgen ray machines, in aircraft engines and electrical devices, especially electric heaters. Small amounts of it are added to copper, aluminum, nickel, cobalt and steel to increase their hardness and resistance to corrosion and high temperatures. Finely powdered beryllium is used as an additive to solid fuel for missiles: Burning coal that contains up to 2.5 ppm of beryllium may constitute an air pollution hazard.

Dr. Waldbott describes a number of cases of what he calls "neighborhood" poisonings by beryllium. Eleven people who lived within two miles of a plant processing beryllium developed the typical symptoms of poisoning. Beryllium dust was found on the clothing of the husband of one of the patients. The coveralls of 100 workers at the plant were tested. The dust shaken out averaged 500 mcg. per meter. Someone in contact with the clothing could inhale 17 mcg. daily of the toxic substance.

In a Pennsylvania refinery and alloy fabricating plant, 26 people living within six miles of the plant had symptoms of beryllium poisoning. Sampling of the air showed 0.105 mcg. per meter, whereas in other parts of the state the levels were only 0.0002 mcg. per meter.

Says Dr. Waldbott, the disease starts insidiously with shortness of breath, weight loss, cough and slight production of phlegm. Sometimes there is fever and nausea. If the interval between exposure to the beryllium and the disease is short, patients often become extremely emaciated and may die within months. As the disease develops, inflammation of the lungs is followed by scarring of the lungs and heart damage. Other organs may be involved as well: liver, kidneys, lymph glands, skin, spleen. And about 40 per cent of patients with chronic beryllium poisoning have high uric acid levels in their blood. This is the condition associated with gout. Beryllium compounds have produced cancers in laboratory animals.

There is what scientists call "synergistic action" between beryllium and a fluoride compound. Hydrogen fluoride in the presence of beryllium sulfate is considerably more dangerous than either one of these compounds by themselves, says Dr. Waldbott.

Adding up exposure to millions of pollutants, one wonders how scientists will ever sort out the cause of some of our disorders.

CHAPTER 22

Nickel

DR. JEAN MAYER, the well known nutritionist of the Harvard University School of Public Health, tells us in his syndicated column for August 23, 1973 that nickel, like chromium, appears to be needed for effective action by certain hormones or gland secretions in the human body. The adrenal glands, which sustain us during stress, and the thyroid gland, which controls many functions, are linked with the nickel in our diets.

Vegetarians have the advantage, it seems, when it comes to nickel, which has now been found to be an essential trace mineral, although no official recommendations have yet been established. There is more nickel in vegetarian products than in foods of animal origin. However, the vegetarian diets must be carefully selected to give ample amounts of unrefined grains and cereal products. Adding oysters would help, too. Plain tea is rich in nickel, as are buckwheat seed and herring.

Most nickel that we ingest is excreted in feces, it appears, since it is poorly absorbed in the digestive tract. Nickel is necessary for several enzyme systems in the body. It is relatively non-toxic, except in enormous doses. Nickel contamination or pollution does not pose any dangerous threat to humans at the present.

According to a report released by the U.S. Department of Agriculture, Agricultural Research Service, North Central Region, Madison, Wis., on June 22, 1973, nickel has been identified as having an essential physiological role in chicks and probably in rats. The research was done at the USDA's Agricultural Research Service Human Nutrition Laboratory at Grand Forks, North Dakota.

"Livers of laboratory animals were adversely affected by deficiency of nickel in their diets," stated Dr. Forrest H. Nielsen, a biochemist, reporting at the 2nd International Symposium on Trace Element Metabolism in Animals. "At present, however, we only have meager insights as to nickel's metabolic function," he said.

The studies were conducted as a preliminary step toward investigations of the possible role of nickel in human nutrition, the USDA said.

Dr. Nielsen and his colleague, Dr. Dwayne Ollerich, professor of anatomy at the University of North Dakota, examined livers from nickel-deprived chicks with an electron microscope and found extensive degeneration of the physical organization of the protoplasm, the USDA continues. Dr. Nielsen consistently observed gross differences—without a microscope—between livers from experimental and control animals. Nickel-deficient chicks' livers were less crumbly and nickel-deficient rats' livers had a muddy brown color compared to a red brown color of livers from their normal counterparts, the scientists reported. The liver, besides secreting bile into the intestines to aid digestion, performs other functions as well. For example, it is involved in building up protoplasm from carbohydrates and proteins.

Dr. Nielsen speculated that further research may show nickel requirements are of greatest importance when there are nutritional diseases caused by diets inadequate in other nutrients.

CHAPTER 23

Cadmium

CADMIUM RED MEDIUM and cadmium orange are two of the most popular oil colors used by painters. Cadmium is a white, ductile, tin-like metal, which some scientists believe is a greater threat to human health than lead, mercury or other heavy metals which are ever-present in our modern technological society.

"At present there does not seem to be any acute risk of chronic cadmium poisoning in the population," reports an editorial in the *Journal of the Norwegian Medical Association*, December 10, 1971, "but what still makes cadmium an important pollutant is its marked tendency to be retained in the body." We apparently dispose of only a small percentage of the cadmium we take in; the rest is stored in the body throughout life.

The American baby has only one microgram of cadmium in his body at birth, but, by the time he is 50, he may have 30 milligrams—30,000 times more than at birth. Dr. James D. Ebert of the Carnegie Institution of Washington, speaking at the 4th International Conference on Birth Defects in Vienna, Austria, September 3, 1973, said that hazards of environmental agents which cause birth defects are so great that development of new screening techniques is essential.

"Man has not evolved means of protecting the embryo against the discoveries of his own laboratories," Dr. Ebert told the conference, which was sponsored by the National Foundation-March of Dimes. "Hence the increasing need for the application of more sophisticated techniques of 'environmental hygiene.'" He added that, since every disease must have both a genetic and an environmental component, it undoubtedly would be easier to remove a defect-causing agent than to alter the action of genes.

Writing in *Environment*, September, 1971, Julian Mc-Caull states that an estimated 2 million pounds of cadmium were released into the atmosphere in 1968 from the tons of scrap melted down in the steelmaking process. More than twice as much cadmium as mercury is used in the United States every year, and one scientist has said, "Cadmium has probably more lethal possibilities than any of the other metals."

Dr. Henry A. Schroeder is quoted in an article, "Trace Pollutants: the Hidden Villains," in the July 21, 1973 issue of *Science News* as saying: "Lead and cadmium are hurting people right now, not because they are highly toxic, but because they are widespread trace pollutants."

Dr. Russell N. Hirst, Jr. of Washington University says in *Medical World News* for September 7, 1973 that, in autopsy studies, he and his associates have found high amounts of cadmium in lung tissue of emphysema patients, and that the severity of the disease is correlated with the amount of cadmium, as well as a history of cigarette smoking. And from Boston University, Dr. Gordon L. Snider and his colleagues report that one cigarette contains about 1 mcg. of cadmium; one pack deposits from 2 to 4 mcg. of cadmium in the smoker's lungs.

Seventy per cent of the cadmium in tobacco passes into the smoke, which is inhaled or goes out into the room to be inhaled by all, smoker and non-smoker alike. Studies of the livers of people dying from emphysema and bronchitis show three times more cadmium than those of people dying of other diseases. Dr. Harold Petering of the University of Cincinnati has shown that the tobacco smoke from one pack of cigarettes, smoked over an 8-hr.

period in a 10- by 12-ft. room, releases over 100 times the amount of cadmium in the outside air.

"Itai, itai!" cried the residents of Kumano Prefecture, Japan, when hundreds of them were afflicted by a disease so painful that even a touch brought the cry (which means "ouch, ouch"). In this condition kidney function is disordered and calcium and other minerals are excreted at a rapid rate. Bones become soft and painful and break easily. There is protein in the urine and also sugar in the urine. Eventually 100 of these agonized sufferers died. Public health officials began to search for the cause of this disaster and they found it: in the river water where a mining and metal company discharged slurry from their mining operations, which was carried downstream to the rice paddies which were irrigated by the river water. Rice grown there was later cooked in the river water. For some 15 years residents of this area had eaten the rice, all the while accumulating cadmium in their bodies. After death the metal was found in high concentrations in their ribs, kidneys and liver. This was one of the earliest indications scientists had of the toxic nature of cadmium, one of the metals being mined on the banks of that Japanese river. In 1955 the company agreed to dam off the polluted water, but soil in the vicinity still carries a heavy load of pollutants.

Dr. Henry Schroeder believes that cadmium has a lot to do with hypertension, or high blood pressure. Analyzing human kidneys obtained at autopsy, he discovered that specimens in Japan, where high blood pressure is prevalent, have twice the cadmium content of the average kidney in the U.S. Kidneys from Africa, where the disease is rare, have less than one-fourth the amount of cadmium in American kidneys. Other countries show the same trend, with cadmium accumulations and high blood pressure following where "civilization" and industrialization are found.

Dr. Schroeder also found that people dying of high

blood pressure had more cadmium in their bodies than those who were not hypertensive. When drugs were used to control the high blood pressure, cadmium levels came down. Raising rats on a diet completely free from cadmium, Dr. Schroeder could find no high blood pressure in them. But as soon as he included in their diet as much cadmium, proportionately, as human beings get, all the females and one-third of the males developed "severe persistent hypertension." He does not believe that cadmium alone is responsible for this rise in blood pressure, nor does he believe it would affect everyone. But it may influence the rising of blood pressure in many people who are susceptible by inheritance.

In *Environment*, October, 1971, Dr. Schroeder elaborated on this theme: "There is little question that cadmium in the air is a real and present hazard to human health. There is good reason to believe that cadmium contributes to high blood pressure in human beings. . . . Concentrations of cadmium in the air and in milk correlate with cardiovascular deaths in the U.S. . . . Cadmium in air is absorbed from the lungs and deposited in the kidney, liver and arteries. It can produce destructive kidney changes and liver damage has been caused by chronic exposure to large amounts. Cadmium is released into the air as a result of incineration or disposal of cadmium-containing products (rubber tires, plastic containers, etc.) and as a by-product in the refining of other metals, primarily zinc."

In one survey, cadmium was detected in 42 per cent of some 720 samples of drinking water from rivers and reservoirs in this country. In addition, the mineral accumulates in water stored in galvanized or plastic water pipes. Phosphate detergents may carry cadmium, along with arsenic, as a pollutant of the phosphates. Refining grains eliminates the zinc which, to some extent, protects us from possible harm from cadmium. So for still another reason, refined and processed foods are not healthful, because the refining of wheat and rice disturbs the relationship between cadmium and zinc. "Areas of the world where the major source of calories is refined grains are apt to show a high incidence of hypertension," says Dr. Schroeder in *Medical World News*, December 23, 1966.

An article in *Science* for May 17, 1963 tells us that when foods were grown in soil heavily fertilized with phosphate they absorbed cadmium. Vegetables normally containing cadmium picked up more of the mineral when the phosphate fertilizer was used—and none in its absence. "Phosphate fertilizers may be a source of the cadmium in some vegetable foods," the article states.

Writing in *Pollution, Profits and Progress*, Dr. Schroeder says, "Without zinc there would be no life. As life evolved during the past 2½ billion years . . . there was so little cadmium around that there was no need to create defense mechanisms against this toxic metal. Man in his infinite wisdom, however, found many uses for cadmium during the last 100 years and has spread it over the globe. But his body has not learned to handle it."

U.S. Public Health Service personnel are investigating the possibility that cadmium may contribute to the many cases of lead poisoning now being found in children in the "inner cities." "Cadmium, much more toxic than lead, is present in trace or even contaminant amounts in old paint," said Dr. Roger S. Challop in the *New England Journal of Medicine*, October 21, 1971. The blood of children who have accumulated too much lead is also loaded with cadmium, says Dr. Challop.

In 1971, Ralph Nader called for studies of the amount of cadmium in gasolines—all gasolines. A California study had found, he said, that four California brands contained cadmium. The cadmium does not come out in the engine exhaust as lead does. Instead, it enters the engine's oils. When these are burned, the cadmium is released as an air pollutant.

The New York Times reported in 1971 that three fish caught near a battery factory on the Hudson River contained up to 1,000 times the normal amount of cadmium. In one nearby cove, said the *Times,* nickel and cadmium deposits are four feet deep. Dr. Henry Schroeder pronounced two of the fish unfit to eat on the basis of their cadmium content; the third was questionable.

In February 1972, Dr. Harriet L. Hardy, a Dartmouth scientist, told an audience at Lafayette College that heart disease and stroke are more widespread in that part of Pennsylvania due to the presence of a huge Bethlehem Steel plant. She noted that the largest single source of cadmium pollution is the melting down of scrap metal to make steel.

At the same symposium, Dr. Robert E. Carroll of the U.S. Public Health Service showed that (using 100 as the average death rate from heart and circulatory diseases) Bethlehem has a 116.5 death rate with 0.021 mcg. of cadmium per cubic meter of air. Philadelphia, with a death rate of 127.6, has 0.023 mcg. of cadmium. Newark, N.J. has a death rate of 119.3 and a cadmium pollution of 0.018. New York City has a death rate of 115.3 and cadmium level of 0.013.

Dr. Carroll added, "Studies have indicated that there is no system or function of the human organism that has not been subjected to and damaged (experimentally or otherwise) by an effective concentration of environmental cadmium." Bethlehem Steel spokesmen said that they do not process scrap at their Bethlehem plant, hence do not put any cadmium into the ambient air.

A June 13, 1973 United Press International story from Palo Alto, Calif. told of two chemists in a scientific instruments measuring concern, who have been measuring amounts of cadmium in various things some of us use every day. Some 15 million pounds of cadmium are used every year in the U.S. for making screws, flashlight batteries, silver solder, bearings, dry cell batteries, etc. Traces of the poison were found in baby foods, tobacco, hair, beverages and countless other items.

In the case of cadmium in food, we should look for foods that contain the least. Foods naturally high in cadmium are coffee and tea, seafood (especially oysters) and canned anchovies. Vegetables and nuts usually contain little cadmium, although we suppose this depends on what kind of fertilizer was used in growing them. Cadmium appears in grains, as we have stated, but it is mostly in the starchy part of the grain. And the zinc in the grain helps to protect us from possible cadmium toxicity.

Don't smoke. Don't sit in rooms where people are smoking if you can avoid it. Don't use the first water that comes out of your water pipes in the morning. Draw water the night before for use in beverages and food for breakfast.

Inquire in your community about the possibility of cadmium air pollution. If you live near a mine or smelter which may be processing one or more of the trace elements associated with cadmium, inquire very thoroughly. Ask the local air pollution officials. They are supposed to know things like this, although, with the current Energy Crisis, some of the standards may have been lowered. If you find that the cadmium content of your air is threatening, write letters to the editor of the local paper and keep others—such as your congressman— informed. With enough public protest you can do a lot toward cleaning up this kind of pollution.

Avoid food in "tin" cans as much as possible. Buy fresh food, organically grown if it is available. Don't burn plastics and try to avoid buying things in plastic containers, since these eventually have to be burned by the local incinerator if they have no other means of disposing of them. Eat unrefined foods, rather than highly processed ones. Shun coffee and tea.

If you want to avoid all minerals in drinking water, drink distilled water. This is not usually recommended, however, unless you have some special health condition which necessitates it. It is generally agreed among scientists that minerals like calcium, magnesium, manganese, lithium and others are healthful when you get them in drinking water.

Many people solve the drinking water problem by buying bottled spring water, which is not very expensive, considering that you use it only for drinking and cooking. However, if you buy bottled spring water, read the label and inquire closely into all the minerals *and trace minerals* the water contains.

Don't be satisfied to know just what levels of calcium, magnesium, sodium, potassium and iron are in the water. Ask about cadmium, lead, arsenic, cyanide. These are some of the trace minerals you want to avoid. There's no sense in paying for bottled water that just might contain more of these undesirable trace minerals than your own community drinking water.

Recently, we inquired about the mineral content of several brands of bottled water. One appeared to be above reproach. It had plenty of calcium, magnesium, iron, potassium, lithium and no objectionable trace minerals were listed. The other company sent us an analysis which showed extremely small amounts of arsenic, cadmium, cyanide, fluoride and lead among other trace minerals. The analysis showed no calcium, magnesium, sodium or potassium, which seems to indicate that this is an analysis only for trace minerals—something which was not included in the analysis of the first brand of water. So there is no way to compare them. The first may be entirely wholesome, but we cannot tell this from the analysis they sent us. The second may contain plenty of the desirable minerals, but we cannot tell that from the analysis they sent us. So we are left in the dark.

If you want to buy bottled spring water, we suggest you get, from the bottler, a complete list of all minerals *and trace minerals* in the water, then send this to the manager of your local waterworks and ask him for his opinion. The U.S. Public Health Service has set permissible levels for most of these minerals by now. These figures should be on file at your local waterworks.

CHAPTER 24

Vanadium

ADDRESSING A 1973 meeting of the American Societies for Experimental Biology, Dr. Leon L. Hopkins, Jr. of the Department of Agriculture stated that "Extrapolating animal data to humans is often misleading. But if man continues to refine and purify his diet without consideration for replenishing extracted trace minerals—such as vanadium—problems that are speculation today may prove to be very real tomorrow."

At a symposium of the American Public Health Association in 1964, Dr. William H. Strain of the School of Medicine and Dentistry, University of Rochester, New York, said, ". . . it is necessary to understand not only how each element functions by itself, but also its relationship to other elements. This is a large task since there are over 70 elements to consider. In general, the availability of each element is variable, the metabolism of all the elements is poorly understood and the interrelationship of elements is only beginning to be studied. Corrective measures include further enriching fertilizers, supplementing animal feeds, and increasing human intake through dietary changes and medication."

He went on to discuss the relationship of vanadium—a light-gray powder with a silvery luster—and zinc. The human body, he said, contains about 1,000 times more zinc than vanadium. But vanadium is important for many purposes in the body. For one, it inhibits the formation of cholesterol in the body. It is a factor in preventing tooth decay. It helps to regulate the way various fats are used. And it is part of the mechanism that surrounds the body's use of two essential amino acids. It should be considered, he says, in its relation to calcium, chromium, cobalt, iodine and manganese.

Vanadium and zinc are important to plant life, and health, and both are present in soil in varying amounts. The amounts which the plants take up from the soil do not necessarily represent the amounts that are there. If there is a lot of vanadium in a certain locality, this is no assurance that all plants grown there will contain lots of vanadium. People who work in plants processing vanadium have lower cholesterol levels than those who do not.

Dr. Strain suggests that one might try lowering his cholesterol level by taking gelatin, which has a rather high content of this mineral. He tells us of a test in which giving 7 grams of gelatin before each meal lowers blood cholesterol, although he says that large-scale trials are necessary before this can be recommended for all of us. One might try it, of course, since gelatin (the unflavored kind) is a good food, valuable for many other reasons as well. For example, it makes some people's fingernails stronger. Keep in mind, when you use gelatin as a source of protein, that it is an incomplete protein and should always be eaten at a meal where some complete protein is available. For example, use milk on your gelatin dessert. Or use hard boiled eggs in your luncheon salad made of gelatin. And, please, remember to use plain gelatin rather than the sugary, dyed, artificially-flavored variety that you find at the supermarket.

Dr. Strain informs us that gelatin from Argentina contains up to 2 ppm of vanadium, whereas that made from American animal bones contains very little—0.1 ppm. "The low vanadium content of gelatin prepared from domestic bones . . . is consistent with the high cholesterol level that is characteristic of civilization," Dr. Strain continues. And he adds that "The extensive use of calcium fertilizers without compensating addition of vanadium may inadvertently be the cause of this decrease in the dietary supply of vanadium throughout the food chain. . . . Our analyses have shown that the vanadium content of hair ranges to 450 parts per billion . . . high blood cholesterol levels are associated with hair vanadium levels of 50 parts per billion or less."

There seems to be no way that human beings ever get too much vanadium and it seems to be non-toxic to humans. Surely Dr. Strain's comments about the inadvisability of using calcium fertilizers containing no vanadium (or other trace minerals) should further reinforce the arguments for organic gardening and against the commercial kind using commercial fertilizers.

An article in *International Journal of Vitamin Research* reports that vanadium content of food is important since it has been found to inhibit or stop off the body's production of cholesterol. We would note that no one is sure whether this is good or bad. There is so much controversy over cholesterol at the moment that, as the election pollsters say, "it's too early to tell" whether too much cholesterol is harmful. Cholesterol is important for many body functions. If you eat lots of cholesterol every day in egg yolk, cream, meat, etc., your body makes less of it. If you are getting very little in food, your body must manufacture more of it. As you remember, cholesterol comes from animal, rather than vegetable, sources.

Vanadium has been found to be related to goiter incidence and tooth decay. Two German scientists report that there are remarkable geographical differences in the vanadium content of drinking water or mineral water. So naturally food cooked in different waters might have widely varying vanadium content.

As with most trace minerals/metals, vanadium is an important industrial commodity. For example, it is used in steel production. Dr. Richard P. Fischer, vanadium commodity geologist of the U. S. Geological Survey, Denver, Colo., speaking at the American Chemical Society's 166th national meeting, August 29, 1973 in Chicago, Ill., said that a shortage of domestic vanadium will develop by the year 2000 and that "mining" petroleum for this important metal was recommended. Fuel oil probably contains more vanadium than any other product of petroleum refining, he said.

"Domestic supplies of vanadium are obtained from a deposit in Arkansas that is mined for vanadium alone, from some deposits in the western states that yield co-product uranium and vanadium, and from slags derived from making elemental phosphorus from phosphate rock mined in Idaho," Dr. Fischer stated. "But the vanadium-production potential of these deposits does not appear to be adequate to satisfy long-range domestic requirements. If the cumulative figures are correct, they show a domestic vanadium deficiency of some 300,000 to 400,000 tons between 1968 and 2000."

CHAPTER 25

Mercury

A SCOTTISH PHYSICIST believes that Charles II died of mercury poisoning. It seems the monarch spent some time in a private laboratory working on a process to distill large quantities of mercury. The researcher recently tested a hair which supposedly came from the head of the king and found it contained 54.6 ppm of mercury. This is about 10 times the amount found recently in some modern people. And it is only a bit lower than the level of mercury which poisoned two workers in a dental lab where mercury poisoning symptoms were clearly evident.

In a similar vein, Prof. James O. Pierce of the University of Missouri Environmental Trace Substances Center, testifying on August 26, 1970 before a Senate Committee in Washington, D. C., said that the Mad Hatter in *Alice in Wonderland* was a victim of mercury poisoning. Mercury was used in the manufacture of felt hats, and it poisons nerves and brains.

In October, 1970, a federal marine biologist discovered that seal liver from the Pribilof Islands—which are in the Bering Sea southwest of Alaska—was heavily contaminated with mercury. What astonished the biologist was that this kind of seal lives in open water 50 to 100 miles from any coastal area. It goes ashore only once a year to mate on the islands. Obviously, the indiscriminate dumping of mercury compounds, DDT, etc., eventually finds its way to the sea, where it enters the food chain from the smallest plankton on up to the largest mammals.

About the same time, the FDA warned expectant mothers not to eat fish taken from waters in several states which are polluted with mercury. In California this meant San Francisco Bay and Delta and some California lakes. In a number of places in Louisiana and Georgia, as well as Lake Erie, mercury has been detected in hazardous levels in some shellfish and commercially caught fish. Dr. Ephraim Kahn, a California Public Health official, stated in *The New York Times*, November 1, 1970, that "mercury has an affinity for the fetus and is much more toxic in unborn children than adults." He referred to studies in Japan showing that mercury poisoning in pregnant women caused their children to be afflicted with mental retardation and cerebral palsy.

In 1971, many newspapers carried headlines about the mercury found in swordfish and tuna. Again, these were some of the largest creatures at the top of the food chain which had gotten large concentrations of mercury by eating smaller fish and other sea life. Dr. Edwin A. Roberts, Jr., a specialist at the oceanographic institute in Woods Hole, Massachusetts, writing in *National Observer*, March 8, 1971, said that for other types of seafood there was little danger from mercury. "Mercury—like lead, arsenic and cadmium—is a very toxic metal that is distributed widely in nature and is harmless in small doses," he said. Five thousand tons of mercury are deposited in the sea every year by soil erosion, but no one has ever come to harm from this, he adds. But man's activities have added an additional 5,000 tons to the seas, and it is this additional burden that worries scientists.

Dr. Roberts says that mercury in waterways becomes toxic only when bacteria in the bottom mud of the sea take it up and change it into methyl mercury, which is absorbed by sea organisms. As we have stated, the metal is taken up first by plankton, which is eaten by tiny fish, which are in turn eaten by larger fish, etc., on to the large predators like tuna and swordfish.

Dr. Roberts notes that 90 per cent of all commercial seeds are treated with mercury compounds to prevent the seeds from being attacked by fungi in the soil before they sprout. So there is a certain residue of mercury in our food grown with this kind of seed. This would be still another reason for favoring organic farming methods.

The *Observer* goes on to give an example of how careless employment of this poison is fairly common. A harbor on Cape Cod (Massachusetts) was closed to shell fishing because of mercury contamination, which scientists suspected came from the greens at a local golf club. A solution which is 73.2 per cent mercury was used to protect the greens, and the residue eventually ran off into the nearby water.

Chemical and Engineering News (February 8, 1971) told the story of a dental assistant who, after her death, was found to have relatively enormous amounts of mercury in kidneys, presumably because she had handled mercury (amalgam) fillings during her 20 years of work. The author, a chemist from England, pointed out that the chief hazard from mercury must be assessed in conjunction with all other environmental pollutants which also attack the nervous system—lead, for example.

Did anybody in your family take calomel as a laxative in the good old days before present-day laxatives were available? It seems that, during the last century, calomel was prescribed by physicians for almost any disorder. Calomel is mercurous chloride, a fairly insoluble form of mercury which, if it is retained in the body for very long, can cause symptoms of mercury poisoning.

Writing in the *Journal of the American Medical Association* for May 24, 1971, Dr. Roy J. Popkin, a California physician, reported: "The pollution of the ocean fish with mercury is a real concern. One source of mercury contamination which appears to have been overlooked, and

I believe should be considered, has been the use of calomel or mercurous chloride in medicine.

"Since the introduction of calomel by Mayerne, a physician to Henry IV of France in the 16th century, it has had a wide use in the treatment of syphilis and as a laxative," Dr. Popkin continues. "It was used in tremendous quantities in the United States in the 19th century. It was the drug of choice for practically every illness known to man. Nineteenth century medical texts list it as the primary drug in such diverse illnesses as fevers, diarrhea, heart disease, worms, rheumatism and eye diseases. Everyone was 'psysicked.'

"The demand for calomel was so great that the pharmacies worked far into the night preparing packages for the next day's demand," Dr. Popkin goes on. "Literally thousands of pounds have been used in this country during the past century, most of it to find its way into the soil, waters and ultimately, the oceans."

Another specialist concerned about the use of calomel is Dr. Larry E. Davis of Johns Hopkins University. He states that "mercurous compounds, widely used in medical preparations and long considered mild and nontoxic may not be so safe as physicians and pharmacists have assumed." Dr. Davis, reporting in *Medical Tribune* for June 20, 1973, states that calomel is still in wide use in laxatives and that the chronic use of such a laxative has been responsible for two deaths. In one case the patient took the laxative daily for 25 years. The other took it for only six years. Both patients showed clear signs of mercury poisoning: unusual timidity, loss of memory, lack of attention, decline of intellect and fine tumors on the hand and face. The two women who died had ominous intestinal and kidney symptoms as well. Brain and nerves also showed extensive damage. "It is our opinion," says Dr. Davis, "that calomel, when taken by mouth, cannot be considered safe."

Drugs in Current Use reports that calomel is not so

widely used as before. If it is used, it should be followed by a saline cathartic, for, if the calomel is not completely eliminated, absorption may occur with resulting systemic mercury reactions.

In *Chemical Week*, January 27, 1971, it is stated that there are 7,000 hospitals in the United States, and that even a small one may dump as much as 150 pounds of mercury a year.

In the April 9, 1974 issue of *The New York Times*, a story appears about mercury pollution which has no special relevance to present mercury contamination in our country. But it tells an insistent and dramatic story of what can happen in respect to trace mineral pollution which is unsuspected and unmonitored. And it reveals impressively the ferocity with which guilty polluters may punish those who expose their depredations or champion their victims.

In the 23 years since the Minamata incident discussed in the article, our environmental pollution specialists have become aware of the ways in which mercury pollution can pose a threat. They now monitor mercury pollution. Ample warning is given of any potential threat. We must insist that these same precautions be taken where there is any chance for danger from trace minerals to this generation or to any generations of the future.

Here is the *Times* article, which was written by Deirdre Carmody:

It is 40 years now since W. Eugene Smith used to dash out of the classroom, clutching his camera, when the great brownish pallor that presages a dust storm would start its sweep across the Kansas sky. In the years since then, his photographs of World War II—recording the bloody invasions of Tarawa, Guam and Iwo Jima—and his intense photo-journalistic essays have ranked him among the greatest living photographers.

In the last two-and-a-half years, Eugene Smith and his Japanese-American wife, Aileen, have been living in the Japanese fishing village of Minamata. They have become passionately involved in exposing and photographing the death and anguish caused by the mercury poisoning of residents who ate fish from the polluted waters there. The Smiths are now completing a book about it.

On July 7, 1972, during the course of a protest against the Chisso Corporation, a chemical company in Minamata that had been dumping industrial waste into the water, Mr. Smith was severely beaten by six men. As a result of his injuries, he is now almost entirely blind.

Two weeks ago his condition worsened considerably. His failing vision disappeared and he was suffused with such violent pain that he kept blacking out.

"The pain is constant," he said the other day. "At the worst of it, I contemplated suicide."

He telephoned from Minamata to Jim Hughes, editor of *Camera 35*, a photography magazine at 132 West 31st Street, which devoted most of its April issue to the photographs and text of Mr. Smith and his wife on the Minamata tragedies.

"Gene called me and told me that he was going blind, that he was desperate, despondent and that he is penniless," Mr. Hughes said.

It was the middle of the night, but Mr. Hughes began telephoning photographers all over the country. He finally reached Lawrence Schiller, a former photographer and now a publisher, who says he has been "very much emotionally moved" by Mr. Smith's work even though he has never met him.

Mr. Schiller called a friend in Tokyo and, although it was then after 2 P.M. on a Friday, the friend made a frantic round of banks and government offices before they closed for the weekend and obtained visas, airplane tickets and money necessary to bring Mr. Smith here for treatment. Then, when it became evident that Mr. Smith could not make the trip to New York alone, Paul Fusco, a photographer and an old friend, flew to Japan from California, went to Minamata and picked up Mr. Smith, then immediately turned around and accompanied him back here.

Mr. Smith is now being treated by Dr. John J. Lalli, an osteopath. As a result of the beating, the vertebrae in Mr. Smith's neck have been jammed together so that they are pinching two nerves and a blood vessel and preventing the flow of blood to his eyes.

In addition, the muscles that control the fingers in his left hand were also affected and he cannot raise his hands high enough to use his camera.

The beating occurred when Mr. Smith, his wife and some of the victims of the poisoning were waiting to see a union leader at the Chisso Company. According to Mr. Smith, he was suddenly surrounded, kicked in the stomach and then slammed across a chair. The six men grabbed his legs and swung him—like a cat, he says—onto the cement courtyard. He landed on his neck as his assailants jumped on him.

He said he did not press charges because he did not want to divert attention from the crusade to get Chisso to concede its moral and financial obligations to the victims. The company newspaper later said that Mr. Smith's injuries were caused by cameras swinging about his neck.

Pain is not new to Mr. Smith, who is now 55 years old. He has survived six plane crashes and a number of battles when he shuttled from invasion to invasion during his wartime coverage for *Life* magazine. He was severely wounded at Okinawa and unable even to pick up a camera for two years thereafter.

Then one day he had the urgent realization that he must get back to work and he became obsessed with the thought that his first photograph should be a success. Painfully, he followed his two children, aged 3 and 5, outdoors and took what was to become perhaps his most famous photograph, "The Walk to Paradise Garden." It shows the children toddling purposefully off into a wooded glen filled with sunlight and it was used as the concluding picture in the "Family of Man" exhibition staged by the Museum of Modern Art in 1955.

Some of his memorable photographs for *Life* include an essay on Welsh miners (1950); life in a primitive Spanish village (1951); a midwife in North Carolina (1951); Dr. Albert Schweitzer and his work in Africa (1954).

In 1955, after he had left *Life*, he began a massive essay on Pittsburgh. "In Pittsburgh, when you could see the moon, it meant poverty because the mines were still and the people were out of work," Mr. Smith recalled the other day. "They were trying to clear up the city so that you could have the moon and prosperity at the same time."

Mr. Smith first went to Minamata, which is on the southern Japanese island of Kyushu, in 1971 with his 21-year-old bride.

"We did not go to take sides, although it became pretty obvious which side we would end up on," he said. "We rented a small place for $9 a month where the first recognized victim of the Minamata disease had lived. It was a child—about five years old—and when she died, they were too poor to bury her. When the money settlement came through later, one of their first acts was to dig up the bones and build a new shrine."

The disease had caused death, brain damage, paralysis, loss of hearing, speech and sight to the bewildered residents of Minamata. It had attacked fetuses in the womb, who were born damaged for life, and there were instances when the mysterious sickness caused by the organic mercury waste impelled humans and animals suddenly to spin into a frenzied dance of death.

The disease, which is now officially called Minamata disease, was first observed in 1951. The dumping was discontinued in 1968, when the old process was replaced by a newer one, and Chisso has since paid a total of $3.6-million to 138 plaintiffs representing 30 families. Mr. Smith contends that there may actually be as many as 10,000 people affected by the disease.

The other day Mr. Smith, who has been profoundly moved by the anguish of Minamata, held up the photograph of a moon-faced, young Japanese girl, who is a victim of the disease, and he read from his forthcoming book:

"Jitsuko-Chan . . . a breathing, haunting, beautiful 19-year-old young lady who will never know a lover. . . . She cannot walk. She cannot talk. It is said if she were to fall into a fire, she would not realize her pain.

"Jitsuko-Chan: no involvement with a human being reacting to their world ever has disturbed me as do you," he read, and as he read, his voice broke.

"That damn beating," he said. "It gets all the publicity and I think it can be used against the Japanese, whom I love.

"But really and truly, all I want is to get my Minamata book done," he said. "None of this stuff about 'dying with his boots on' or 'He was a photographer until his dying day.' We just must finish that book."

"Beginning in early September 1971, almost 100,000 metric tons of fungicide-treated wheat and barley, intended exclusively for seed use, were distributed to farmers of rural Iraq," reports *Science News*, July 21, 1973. "Unable to read or understand printed warnings on the sacks, many villagers began to make flour and homemade bread from the grains and ingested around 1.4 mg. of methyl mercury per loaf eaten. Within a few months 6,530 cases of mercury poisoning were admitted to hospitals, where 459 of the patients died.

"When body concentration of the chemical rose to between 20 and 40 mg., first symptoms of toxicity began to appear, mainly numbness and loss of coordination. Death occurred at about 200 mg. Unborn children proved most susceptible, often having higher concentrations of mercury than their mothers at birth and suffering severe brain damage if they survived."

The authors, who made their initial report in the July 20, 1973 issue of *Science*, recommended further studies to find what can be done to help future victims and determine what levels of the much publicized mercury contamination in fish can be considered safe for human consumption.

Keep in mind that the individual whose resistance is low in every way will be an easier victim for poisons of all kinds. Watch your diet, take your food supplements, get your exercise, get plenty of sleep. Be the Ralph Nader on your block and take up your new hobby with gusto—pollution fighting!

CHAPTER 26

Lead

In 1792, one of the world's most famous and talented painters, Francisco de Goya, fell ill of a disease which all but killed the 46-year-old man. He was incapacitated for more than a year. His symptoms were paralysis of the right side, vertigo or dizziness, impairment of balance, hearing and speech, partial blindness, convulsions, mental confusion, hallucinations and periods of coma. This would account for the grotesque paintings of this period that hang in the Prado Museum in Madrid. Finally, he had to stop painting. After a year away from his studio, he recovered, except for permanent deafness.

A New York psychiatrist was quoted in *The New York Times* for February 8, 1972 as saying he believes that Goya's illness was lead poisoning, due to his methods of work. He used enormous amounts of white paint, which he mixed himself from a highly toxic compound containing lead carbonate. He worked with great rapidity, often completing a painting in several days. He threw his lead-based paint around with abandon, using sponges, mops rags to apply it to the canvasses. In the process he could have absorbed into his blood many times the "safe" amount of lead vapors. The terrible nervous symptoms which resulted disappeared after he had been away from painting for a year. Although there were many unhappy episodes in his life, the illness no doubt affected the quality and subject matter of his pictures during this period.

Today, in cities around the world, studies are being made of lead poisoning and threats of lead poisoning in homes where old lead-based paint has flaked from the walls. Slum children, cooped up all day inside with nothing much to do, often eat the lead flakes. A recent study involved 27 cities in 23 states. In 85 per cent of them dangerous amounts of flaking lead paint were found. The investigators tested 2,309 children living in these old houses and found that almost 10 per cent have blood levels of lead above what the FDA authorities believe is "safe." One or two of these children had the classic symptoms of lead poisoning. In others those symptoms are possibly still to come. This study was reported in the June 21, 1973 issue of *Medical Tribune*.

The Food and Drug Administration has banned the manufacture of high-lead paints (this was after December, 1972), over the protests of the paint industry. The allowable levels are only 0.5 per cent of lead. It is worthy of note that the Federal Department of Housing and Development has exempted itself from this ban on lead paint in new housing that is now under construction. Much of this, of course, would be housing for the children who are now risking lead poisoning in their old tumbledown homes. And almost nothing is being done to remove the old lead paint which is the real hazard.

Meanwhile, authorities are finding many children with raised blood levels of lead who do not live in slum houses or eat flaked paint. *Chemical and Engineering News* for February 14, 1972, in its letters to the editor column, states the probable reason: lead in the air of cities from leaded gasoline. The letter, signed by the Graduate Class in Environmental Chemistry, Loyola University, points out that measuring just the lead in the air does not give a true picture. When the air pollution stirred up in big city traffic settles to the ground, the dust may contain up to 6 per cent lead by weight—60,000 ppm—far, far more than any allowable levels of this highly toxic substance.

Every chemist is taught that lead salts are toxic. Every chemist is aware that tetraethyl lead is added to gasoline. So why have we allowed this situation to develop? the graduate students ask.

"A few months ago," states *Science News*, July 21, 1973, "the Environmental Protection Agency reported over a fourth of all American children have levels of lead in their bodies that border on toxicity."

A report by the National Academy of Sciences on airborne lead, released in 1971, brought accusations of bias in understating the hazards of the lead which city dwellers breathe daily. One of the authorities whose work formed the basis of the report has worked for the Ethyl Corporation for more than 50 years. Protesting against this kind of "research," one scientist from City University of New York said, in *Science*, July 7, 1972: "In my long career in the field of public health, with emphasis on occupational health and air pollution, I have been witness to the biases of industrially employed experts a great many times. . . . It is pure naivete for the National Academy of Sciences . . . not to recognize such facts. It is foolhardy to ask any biased scientist to interpret facts, the explanation of which may be variable, without taking into consideration his biases."

Of the 18 tons of lead deposited daily on Los Angeles, most is immobile, apparently accumulating, except for the 4.3-ton dose blown daily into adjacent areas, Dr. J. J. Huntzicker and Dr. S. K. Friedlander of the California Institute of Technology told the 166th national meeting of the American Chemical Society, Chicago, Ill., August 29, 1973.

Current fallout measurements show that 2.1 tons of airborne lead descend each day upon urban Los Angeles and another 0.4 tons fall into coastal waters, the scientists and a graduate student, Cliff I. Davidson, said. A different type of measurement showed that about 10 tons of lead per day are deposited directly on or near the roadways of metropolitan Los Angeles. About 75 per cent of lead additives in gasoline are emitted into the air, they explained.

Vegetables grown alongside superhighways in our country have been found to contain 50 times more lead than the amount considered tolerable in food. They pick it up from the exhaust of cars and trucks. Says *New Scientist* for December 5, 1963, "Countless people may be regularly swallowing minute amounts but dangerous quantites of poisonous metallic elements. But this is not only because man is busily poisoning his environment, but also because feeding growing populations means huge quantities of food are now being grown or reared on land never before used for the purpose and which may contain harmful substances."

Prof. Harry V. Warren of the University of British Columbia, in a meeting on trace minerals pointed out that, in one county in England some of the people have "Derbyshire neck"—a goiter due to lack of iodine—and some have "Derbyshire tummy"—a colic resulting from too much lead in their food and water. Dr. Warren believes that lead in our environment may be related to incidence of multiple sclerosis. In 24 localities he studied where MS incidence was high, there were also high levels of lead in rocks and soils. In other areas where MS was below average, there was average or lower content of lead.

Still other sources of lead are turning up all the time. An August 13, 1972 release from the College of Medicine and Dentistry of New Jersey noted that many children chew on bits of newspaper or magazine. Printer's ink contains large amounts of lead. Such children may be getting far too much for their own good. And what happens to the lead when city incinerators burn newspapers and magazines? Well, it floats off into the air and adds to the already heavy burden of lead pollution caused by traffic.

In spite of official warnings on lead-based pottery, some companies are still selling it. Recently an enterprising housewife who leads a Rochester, New York consumer group asked her local health authorities to test a brand of pottery being sold in local stores. They found that the dishes would leach 155 ppm of lead into any food stored in them for any length of time. The company recalled the pottery from local stores but refused to issue a warning to people who had already bought it.

The New England Journal of Medicine reported (September 24, 1970) on two cases of children poisoned by drinking fruit juice from a modern, handmade earthenware jug. One of the children died. Testing other kinds of pottery, officials found that of 264 earthenware dishes, 50 per cent released enough lead to make them unsafe for cooking or storing food. Up to 25 per cent of these were capable of causing severe lead poisoning.

As if it weren't enough that you have to worry about all the chemicals in toothpaste—fluoride, for example—we find that there may be lead in the toothpaste as well. E. Berman, writing in *Archives of Environmental Health* (July, 1972), gives the results of tests of 18 popular brands of toothpaste. Three were found to contain potentially hazardous amounts of lead. A University of Pennsylvania research team says that you should definitely not squeeze the tube to get the last drop. Reporting in the *Journal of the American Dental Association* (February, 1973), they tested six commercial brands of toothpaste and found that the paste from the end of the tubes contained from 4 to 72 times as much lead as paste from inside the tube.

The FDA now claims that all toothpaste tubes are now made of plastic and aluminum. It seems that the fluoride used in some of the toothpaste necessitated a lead tube.

In July, 1972, a Boston health official told the press that a considerable amount of lead may be eroding from the surface of lead water pipes and getting into the drinking water of Boston and possibly other cities. Dr. Dorothy Worth said: "Lead piping is still in wide use throughout the U.S., and anywhere you have lead pipe and corrosive water, you could have lead poisoning." And a 1969 report in *Lancet* shows that bones of people who have lived in a "soft" water area contain more lead than those in "hard" water areas. The soft water may leach out more lead from the pipes than hard water does. *Today's Health* of several years ago stated that lead water pipes connecting home plumbing to the local water main might result in lead poisoning. Symptoms may be gradual and not be apparent for years, the magazine said. Children are more likely to be affected than adults.

Some experts in the field of trace minerals believe that the Romans may have lost their empire because of lead poisoning. The Romans kept their food, wine and other beverages in lead vessels. As we have just reported, lead-based dishes and utensils can be dangerous. The most recent incident involves antique pewter salt shakers. In earlier times, tin and lead were the main constituents of pewter; today it is mostly tin. At any rate, a woman came to a hospital complaining of nine months of severe abdominal pain, progressive profound weakness, loss of appetite and weight. She had been using lots of salt daily from the antique pewter shakers. Doctors examined the shakers and found 20 micrograms of lead per 10 grams of salt when the shakers were used for one hour. They treated the woman with a chelating agent which removes lead from the body.

In several parts of the country airborne lead from industrial plants threatens the health of children living near. Dr. Henry Schroeder has stated, "Evidence of a biochemical abnormality in persons exposed to urban air concentrations of lead is beginning to appear. There is little doubt that, at the present rate of pollution, diseases due to lead toxicity will emerge within a few years."

Dr. Robert A. Kehoe of the University of Cincinnati

Kettering Laboratories says there is some lead in all food that we eat. He puts the average daily consumption at 0.3 milligrams. Sea bass caught off Los Angeles recently contained 22 ppm of lead in their livers, perhaps two or three times the "normal" amount.

The National Air Pollution Control Administration estimates that 200,000 tons of lead are added to the atmosphere each year and 95 per cent of this is from automobile exhausts.

A survey of the neighborhood where the New York upper income children with high lead concentrations live disclosed that there are in the area two auto shops which spray-paint cars, a wrought-iron works that uses lead paint, an artist's paint factory, several typesetting shops. The West Side Highway is a few blocks away. This is an elevated highway where cars move bumper to bumper most of the day and night.

As you move farther away from main highways, the lead content of blood decreases. The lead content of Arctic ice increased four-fold from 1750 to 1940, but nearly tripled between 1940 and 1965. The Antarctic, much farther away from the industrial northern hemisphere, shows only one-tenth the lead of the Arctic.

A Siberian tiger at the Philadelphia Zoo died of lung cancer. Authorities at the zoo said that, until 1935, there was only one case of lung cancer among the birds in the zoo. Since 1935 they have had 15 deaths, mainly among those water birds which are outside on the lake. There is a similar rise in lung cancer among all animals which live outside. Those inside appear to be relatively free of lung cancer. Apes and monkeys, kept inside glass cages with little polluted air entering, are free from lung cancer. The Philadelphia zoo is surrounded by thruways, with hundreds of thousands of cars racing past all sides of the zoo all day.

Prof. Sumner M. Kalman of Stanford University School of Medicine says: "We have not begun to appreciate what the fate of automobile lead will be. We haven't begun to uncover the Pandora's box of tricks that nature has in store for us. . . . We are nowhere near as smart as the petroleum people think we are." He points out that people who have difficulties with blood disorders are especially at risk, since lead attaches itself to the red blood corpuscles in the body. Since it interferes with the manufacture of hemoglobin, the red coloring matter of blood, it may produce anemia. A high level of calcium in the diet protects to some extent against the possibility of lead poisoning, according to a news release from Cornell University in August, 1973.

Some babies are born with lead levels in their blood of 0.02 milligrams per cent. Their mothers, according to the survey, showed the same concentrations. If these children go out into a world where lead pollution stalks them, is it not possible that they will be "quickly poisoned?" asks Dr. Shrihari Sakhadeo of Montefiore Hospital in New York City.

On November 6, 1972, *The New York Times* published a four-paragraph article stating that "significant amounts of lead" have been found in evaporated milk. The lead has apparently leached from the lead material which is used to seal the can. This metal may be as much as 50 per cent lead. New York officials found that 13-oz. cans of evaporated milk contained as much as 1,200 mcg. of lead. Only 300 mcg. are considered as permissible intake *from all sources,* according to Dr. Vincent Guinee. The 11 leading manufacturers of evaporated milk whose products were tested could not be reached for comment. The city has told them that corrective action must be taken, the *Times* says.

The New York State Health Department, on May 15, 1973, reported that it had found "undesirable levels" of lead in a variety of baby foods and other foods packaged in lead-soldered cans. "Dr. Hollis S. Ingraham, the state Health Commissioner, said he was asking the FDA to open a 'further investigation' because researchers found 100 parts per billion or more of lead in 70 per cent of 155 lead-seam cans tested," states *The New York Times*, May 16, 1973.

"The FDA now considers 500 parts a billion an acceptable lead level in any product that is later diluted, like evaporated milk. There are no standards yet for full-strength products like juice. The state said that 20 per cent of the lead-seam cans it tested contained 400 or more parts a billion," the *Times* continues. "If a child drank a pint of liquid with 300 parts a billion lead in it, the child would be approaching the danger point in lead ingestion—the point at which it begins to accumulate at a significant rate in the body rather than be expelled. This kind of accumulation increases the risk of lead poisoning, the state said."

The FDA to date has not taken any action on the lead in canned milk, despite an announcement that they would issue regulations in January, 1973. No regulations for canned juices for babies have been announced either.

An article in the October 28, 1972 *Lancet* should come as no surprise. Three New York psychiatrists reported on a study of lead in the blood of hyperactive children. They found that hyperactive children have raised levels of lead in their blood. More than half of those studied had levels classified as "raised" but not toxic. Giving the hyperactive children a compound which causes the body to excrete lead, they found in the urine of 60 per cent levels of lead that were in the "toxic" range. The authors say that large amounts of lead in the body may have results which were hitherto unrealized. They believe that physicians should look for raised levels of lead in all children who demonstrate hyperactive activity, that is, they are fidgety, they daydream a lot, they skip school, they are sometimes unruly.

"Is lead blowing our minds?" asks the title of an article in *New Scientist*, May 27, 1971. A University of Reading,

England, professor believes that lead pollution from automobiles may be responsible for a significant proportion of mental illness. As we have shown, lead is a cumulative poison which stops the activity of certain enzymes and tends to replace calcium in bones. Admissions to mental hospitals in England showed an increase of 11 per cent in all ages between 1964 and 1968. But admissions of girls under 10 have gone up 100 per cent and those of boys under 10 have gone up 60 per cent.

Jon Tinker, the very knowledgeable writer of the *New Scientist* article, points out that, for some kinds of pollution which affects only a few people, where levels of exposure are substantially lower than those known to be toxic, where the symptoms of poisoning are easily recognized and where the pollution comes from some activity that is absolutely essential, then it seems worthwhile to take some risk. But "where whole populations are exposed to levels close to the toxic thresholds, where symptoms are hard to identify and poisoning is irreversible, where pollution can be avoided at moderate inconvenience and cost—then the risk is in no way worth running. For lead, the case for playing safe is gradually becoming overwhelming."

In adults, early symptoms of lead poisoning include fatigue, sleep disturbance and constipation. In children, permanent brain damage can result which leads to mental retardation, irritability, abnormal behavior patterns that are similar to manic-depressive illness. Residents of a Swiss city complained of these symptoms, and were given chelation treatments which causes the individual to excrete heavy metals from the blood. Sixty-five per cent showed complete improvement; 20 per cent partial improvement.

When newborn rats were suckled by mothers eating a diet containing 4 per cent lead, they became hyperactive at four weeks of age, reports the December 8, 1973 issue of *Science News*. There was an 8-fold increase in lead in their brains, and a 20 per cent decrease in the nerve chemical dopamine, suggesting that lead can upset dopamine and in turn the central nervous system, reported Dr. Mitchell W. Sauerhoff and Dr. I. Arthur Michaelson of the University of Cincinnati.

Dr. Ellen Silbergeld and Dr. Alan M. Goldberg of the Johns Hopkins University School of Public Health also found that lead poisoning can lead to hyperactivity in mice. Their report was made October 2, 1973 at the Conference on Low Levels of Lead Toxicity in Raleigh, North Carolina. They reported that chronic ingestion of lead can produce a significantly increased level of motor activity in mice, which strengthens the evidence that a similar link exists between lead poisoning and minimal brain dysfunction, or hyperactivity, in children. This research is discussed in more detail in a December 10, 1973 press release from the National Institutes of Health, Washington, D.C.

This all sounds as though things have gotten out of hand insofar as environmental lead is concerned, wouldn't you agree? What can you do to protect yourself and your family? Obviously, the first step is to make certain there are no walls with flaking paint anywhere in your neighborhood. When you buy paint, make certain that its lead content, if any, is 0.5 per cent or lower.

Avoid heavily traveled streets and, if possible, see that your children do not walk or play on such streets. Don't take the car out at times when traffic is heavy. With the Energy Crisis you should be using public transportation anyway, in areas where it is available. If you must drive, arrange your working hours so that you will avoid traffic jams. Buy unleaded gasoline and ask your friends to do likewise. Write to Detroit, to the makers of your car, and tell them how you feel about city air pollution and the enormous role of the automobile motor in this pollution.

Don't store food in any earthenware containers. Many times, however, it is impossible to check whether there is lead in the glaze. Don't buy evaporated milk until the lead-seam can situation is cleared up. Call your city waterworks and inquire if lead pipes bring the water from its source into local homes. If so, ask them if the lead content of the water has been tested. If it is high, protest. And buy bottled water for drinking and cooking.

But, as we have shown, the most significant danger from lead pollution is the same dilemma that faces us with all environmental pollution. The damage is cumulative. If you are exposed to only one or two sources of minimal lead pollution, it may be harmless. But if there are many sources to contend with, your body suffers from this accumulated stress.

Would you like to know how much of the trace minerals you have in your body—both the helpful and harmful ones? The Soil and Health Foundation, a non-profit organization, can arrange to have tests (hair analysis of trace minerals) made for members at a moderate cost. To become a member, send a contribution of any amount to The Soil and Health Foundation, Emmaus, Pa. 18049. Request information on the hair test service. In addition to the membership contribution, there is an extra charge for the hair analysis.

CHAPTER 27

Other Trace Minerals

HERE IS A brief summary on the potential hazards or benefits of some of the lesser known trace minerals. It is well to keep in mind that there is disagreement among authorities on some of these statements. As research in trace minerals is accelerated, no doubt more of the riddles will be solved.

Aluminum. This metal occurs in the human body and in the bodies of animals which have never eaten food prepared in aluminum utensils; minute amounts of it, too, may be essential, writes Adelle Davis in *Let's Eat Right to Keep Fit.*

Dr. Schroeder says that aluminum poses no problem in pots and pans and is, in fact, probably inert. It is a major problem in beer can litter along our roadsides, as all environmentally aware people know. This poses one of the most troublesome problems so far as solid waste disposal is concerned.

Dr. Underwood also believes that aluminum pots and pans and aluminum-containing baking powder pose no threat to human health. He reports that 10 times the amounts we might get in this way can be handled by the human body. There are, of course, people who feel that aluminum utensils should not be used. If you are one of these, then by all means get rid of your aluminum things. But, when you are contemplating their possible toxicity, keep in mind Dr. Schroeder's warning about the potential harm that may reside in "tin" cans which, he says, contain traces of just about every mineral present in junked cars. A recent study *(International Journal for Vitamin and Nutrition Research,* Vol. 43, 1973) gives estimates of aluminum content of the human diet as varying between 5 and 135 mg. daily.

Antimony is toxic. It is present in some ceramics and glazes. People have been poisoned by exposure to antimony in polluted food. It is also used in toothpaste tubes, solder, ammunition, fireworks, matches, pigments, plastics, rubber or type metal. You see what our modern industrialized civilization can do when it really sets its mind to spreading some of these toxic substances around the planet in all kinds of gadgets and trinkets.

Arsenic. It's not toxic in small amounts, although it does cause skin problems and cancer in moderate amounts and in larger amounts it is a killer poison. If you don't think so, find out what Abbey Brewster and her sister did to those homeless old men in Joseph Kesselring's play, *Arsenic And Old Lace.* Arsenic is used in herbicides, pesticides, wood preservatives, rat poisons and cotton-growing. We should worry about high levels of this mineral in drinking water. In areas where phosphate-rich detergents are washed into waterways, the arsenic they contain goes right along into the water.

For some reason chickens and pigs grow better and thrive when a small amount of arsenic is included in their diets. It is believed that the arsenic has somewhat the same effect as antibiotics in digestive tracts, preventing infections, we suppose. If you are on the mailing list of the FDA, you will get through the mail long lists of additives permitted in the feed of poultry and animals. It is always a shock to find arsenic listed there. The organic poultryman or stock farmer does not use this additive.

On December 12, 1972, the U.S. Department of Agriculture stated that almost one out of every six chicken livers are contaminated with illegal residues of organic arsenic. The USDA also said that 1.7 per cent of the nation's pork livers showed illegal amounts of organic arsenic during random sampling tests. A spokesman at the USDA's Animal and Plant Health Inspection Service in Washington, D.C., said that the organic form of arsenic, used to stimulate growth, "is not particularly dangerous to humans in quantities found in the samples," reported the *New York Post*.

Barium is only slightly toxic, according to Dr. Schroeder. It is added to diesel fuel to suppress smoke. Barium is the radioactive substance doctors give you to swallow when they take X-rays of your digestive tract. It is also used in glass, paint, rubber, ceramics, plastics, road flares, fireworks, sugar refining, says Dr. Schroeder. It occurs to us that the ever-present pollution of everything near a heavily traveled highway might include barium from the rubber flakes from tires. A recent news item from Philadelphia tells us that tiny, microscopic mists of rubber particles are present in enormous numbers in the Philadelphia air, due probably to the stuff that is shredded off tires along heavily traveled roads. The Air Management Services spokesman suggested washing the streets oftener to keep the rubber particles from blowing up into the air.

Bismuth is in antacids and steel products. In these preparations it is insoluble and hence harmless, says Dr. Schroeder. But when it appears in cosmetics—"white" lipsticks, body powders and medicines—no one knows what its potential for harm may be. It should be watched, he believes.

Drugs in Current Use reports that some compounds of bismuth may be given for mechanical protection of the skin or digestive tract. Often used for diarrhea, it is insoluble and hopefully harmless. Other bismuth compounds, however, were used against syphilis when arsenic was also being used to treat this disease. Bismuth given internally may cause toxic effects: skin eruptions, inflammation of the mouth and kidney irritation.

Boron is used in glass, soaps, cleansers, porcelains, fiberglass, glass wool, tanning, adhesives and starch manufacture. Boric acid has been used as a mild external germicide for many years but, strangely, nobody has ever done much research on its potential toxicity. We know boron best from borax and boric acid; borax is the way this element appears as an ore in nature. It has been known and used since prehistoric times. When applied in excess, however, or when taken internally, boric acid can kill. There have been instances when infants have been given boric acid rather than sugar in their formulas, by mistake of course, and results have been fatal. There seems to be no evidence that boron is needed by either animals or man.

A study of the amount of boron in food was reported in the *International Journal for Vitamin Research*, Vol. 43, 1973. Two German scientists report that they found astonishing differences in boron content of food—variations from 0.3 to 41 mg., depending chiefly on where the foods were grown; that is, the geographical location. The authors say that this raises questions about the possibility of getting too much in some areas, since boron is also used as an additive in some instances.

Germanium apparently occurs in our diets at the rate of about 1½ mg. per day. It is rapidly and apparently harmlessly excreted. It appears to be non toxic to both animals and man.

Palladium causes cancer in mice. We human beings have very little exposure to it. It is in the family of platinum and is very rare.

Radium is the famous radioactive element with the extremely long half-life of 1,620 years. Because of the precautions taken, radium poisoning is rare. This element was discovered in 1898 by Madame Curie and her husband. Radium therapy is often used to treat certain diseases.

Rhodium is used to electroplate microscopes and instruments. It is in the platinum group and human exposure to it is very low, which is fortunate, since it causes cancer in mice.

Rubidium is closely related to potassium, as is *cesium*, another trace mineral. There is some evidence that rubidium might act as a substitute for potassium in some physiological activities. Plant foods contain about 35 ppm of rubidium, the cereal grains a bit less, and white flour much less.

Silicon is just about everywhere in the environment. It represents some 28 per cent of the earth's crust. It is a non-metallic element which occurs in plants, animals and human beings. In the human, silicon is rapidly eliminated through the urine. As an air pollutant, it is extremely dangerous to the lungs of miners and stoneworkers, causing silicosis. Dr. Underwood tells us that the amount of bone ash of baby rats on a low-calcium diet is influenced by the amount of silicon in their diets and the amount of silicon in their bones is influenced by the amount of calcium as well as silicon in their diets.

Scientists at the 1973 meeting of the American Societies for Experimental Biology reported that silicon has now been found to be essential for good health. It is involved in forming cartilage. Dr. Edith M. Carlisle of the University of California at Los Angeles said she had found that tissues rich in silicon are connective tissues and cartilage, as in the trachea, the aorta, the skin and the eyes. It's significant that in aging there is a great decrease in the silicon content of the aorta of rats, chicks and rabbits. The aorta is the major blood vessel of the heart. It decreases in the skin, too, and there is a tremendous drop in silicon in the thymus; in old animals there's about 2 ppm, compared with 56 ppm in young ones.

Silver, of course, is used for all kinds of things and is generally inert and insoluble. It is used in medicine for caustic, astringent and antiseptic purposes. Mostly we know it as the silver nitrate put in newborn babies' eyes to prevent possible blindness caused by gonorrhea. Silver preparations tend to stain the skin, so lengthy application of any silver medications on skin or mucous membranes or taking small doses internally may cause permanent bluish discoloration of the skin which is called *argyria.* Silver salts in large amounts are potent poisons, affecting the nervous system or the digestive tract and causing convulsions, paralysis, depression of vital centers or gastroenteritis. There is apparently no way that such disasters could afflict any of us as a result of environmental contamination.

Strontium is built into bones and teeth. It may help to prevent tooth decay and broken bones in older people. Much of it is removed when grains are refined. Strontium 90 is the radioactive form of this mineral which floated down through the air during the bomb-testing of the past decades. Since its half-life is 28 years, we can assume that most of this radioactive pollution has disappeared by now, causing us no further concern until somebody gets the idea of shooting off more nuclear bombs.

Sulfur is found in proteins: eggs, milk, fish, poultry. It does not exist in carbohydrate or fat. Three of the essential amino acids contain sulfur. Two vitamins—thiamine (B1) and biotin, also a B vitamin—contain sulfur. This yellowish substance is used in making gunpowder, matches, medicines and in vulcanizing rubber.

Since there appears to be no chance that anyone eating a diet that will sustain life will be short on sulfur (it is so widespread in foods), the only concern we may have about it is that it is especially important because it occurs in the amino acid methionine. Vegetarian diets tend to be short on this amino acid.

Tellurium is obtained chiefly as a by-product in the

refining of copper and lead. It is toxic to workers who are exposed to it. It is found, says Dr. Schroeder, in "tin" cans. Should we worry about it? Who knows?

Tin appears to collect more readily in tissues of people in the industrialized part of the world, while in Africa there is little accumulation. Supposedly we Americans take in up to 3½ mg. daily if we regularly eat food from cans. It has been established that the person who eats a diet of mostly fresh foods like meat, vegetables and grain products might get as little as 1 mg. a day, while people who eat substantial portions of canned vegetables and fish might get as much as 38 mg. a day. Most cans these days are lacquered, which prevents much of the contamination with tin, but even so, canned food stored for some time can pick up considerable tin due to defects in the lacquer. It seems possible that we people in the industrialized world get most of our tin from canned foods. It has low toxicity, apparently, and is excreted readily in urine and feces.

Reporting on the essential nature of tin at a meeting of the Federation of American Societies for Experimental Biology, Dr. Klaus Schwarz of Long Beach, California VA hospital, said: "Tin had been disqualified as an essential trace element because it couldn't be found in newborn infants. But it's necessary at a level of 1 to 2 ppm in the diet—that much tin can be found in many plant and animal nutrients."

According to Dr. Jean Mayer of Harvard University, it has now been discovered that tin is needed for health in laboratory animals. They won't grow without it. "Extra tin in normally fed healthy animals does not produce supergrowth, however," says Dr. Mayer, "so there is no point in would-be basketball players starting to gnaw on the family's discarded tin cans."

Titanium is used in paints, sunburn cream and in certain alloys to impart toughness. It is like aluminum, very abundant in the earth's crust and in soils, but poorly absorbed by plants and animals. Most of the titanium that occurs in foods is believed to be the result of contamination. Titanium in the lungs appears to come from air pollution. No one has yet discovered that this element is essential in any way for animals or human beings.

Uranium is slightly radioactive and is used in nuclear reactors. Uranium 235 may be made to undergo nuclear fission with the release of large amounts of energy. Uranium 238, another isotope, can absorb a neutron to produce Uranium 239. This spontaneously loses a beta particle of radiation to form *plutonium*. There is nothing you need be concerned about in all this complex situation until you are faced with a nuclear power plant in your area, at which time you will have to become very familiar with all the radioactive isotopes and their potential harm to human beings. Plutonium, derived from uranium, is the single most toxic material in the world, according to nuclear physicists. The Atomic Energy Commission and the electric power industry are planning to use it in comparatively large amounts in their nuclear power program. With a half-life of 24,000 years, plutonium is by far the most deadly of all the worrisome nuclear trinkets we discovered inside the Pandora's box of nuclear fission.

Zirconium resembles titanium and silicon. It is used in flints for cigarette lighters and in antiperspirants, which can cause skin irritation. It has been found in many human tissues and its accumulation there exceeds that of some other trace minerals—copper, for example. We get, supposedly, about 3½ mg. daily, chiefly from meat, dairy foods, vegetables, cereals and nuts. There is no evidence that zirconium is harmful and also no evidence that we need it.

CHAPTER 28

Why We Recommend
Organic Farming
and Gardening

THE UNITED STATES Department of Agriculture, which is continuously engaged in downgrading and belittling organic farming and all the principles which underline it, publishes each year a *Yearbook*, which we have quoted in this book. In 1959 the annual was devoted to *Food*. Here are some assorted quotes having to do with minerals and trace minerals in the soil.

"One of the most important of the many variables in the soil is the supply of available mineral nutrients the plants need for growth."

"The regional differences in the mineral content of soils may or may not be reflected in the levels of the minerals in plants. . . ."

"The absorption of mineral ions by plant roots is a complicated process. All the facts needed for an adequate explanation are not yet known. Soil structure, pH (acidity), soil microorganisms and moisture exert an influence on this process. . . ."

"Some places in the country are deficient in minerals. The mineral content of the soil there is reflected in the low mineral levels of the plants. Thus, copper deficiency areas exist in the Southeast, notably Florida, and cattle pastured there must receive additional copper. . . ."

"Fertilizers can be improperly used, of course, and the organic aspects of soils can be—and generally are—badly neglected in this country. . . ."

This is precisely what organic gardeners and farmers have been saying. We wish that some of the arrogant diehards in the USDA and FDA who belittle organic farming techniques would go back and read the 1959 yearbook, along with more recent material on the subject.

Trace mineral deficiencies are now reported in 50 states, with major areas of depletion as follows: zinc deficient in the soils of 43; boron in 41; manganese in 30; molybdenum in 27; iron in 25; copper in 14. This information was reported in *Farm Chemicals*, February 1967.

Just how much of the various trace minerals are in the soil of your garden or the garden or farm where your food is grown? Here is a chart from a report in *Science* for April 23, 1965. It shows the amount of nine trace minerals in the soil of a garden in Maryland, a forest in Maryland, a garden in New York, a garden in New Mexico and an area of "natural soil" in the same state. It also shows the trace mineral content of worldwide soil. As you can see, there are wide differences from state to state and in localities in that state. These figures were published in 1953. We do not know what changes there have been since then. The figures are given in ppm.

Element	Mary-land Garden	Forest	N.Y. Garden	N. Mexico Garden	Nat. soil	World-wide Soil
Iron	40,000	47,000	19,000	30,000	20,000	38,000
Manganese	1,200	1,400	620	700	400	850
Tin	6,000	5,500	4,000	5,000	3,500	4,600
Chromium	70	70	60	30	45	200
Nickel	30	30	30	15	10	40
Arsenic	19	8	11	14	9	5
Lead	150	25	420	70	18	10
Copper	100	65	100	25	28	20
Zinc	100	35	240	80	40	50

Iron, manganese, copper and zinc are gaining more respect in the field of nutrition as studies of human diseases link imbalances of these elements to various disorders, according to an article in *Organic Marketing* for June, 1973.

"A series of experiments . . . were conducted by Drs. Robert F. Keefer and Rabindar N. Singh of West Virginia University's Agricultural Experiment Station. Tests with sweet corn and field corn revealed that the kinds and amounts of fertilizers used on soil can cause changes in the trace elements of the final product," the article reports. Such a finding surely indicates that serious consequences may follow the almost universal American practice of using commercial fertilizers which, in general, contain only three minerals (calcium, phosphorus and potassium) and neglect entirely all the trace minerals.

"Because of the minute amounts of these trace elements found in food and in the human body, their nutritional significance has only recently been recognized," the article continues. Sweet corn grains, for instance, contain an average of only 114 ppm of iron, the researchers point out.

"Recent medical findings, however, which have implicated zinc deficiency in man with an iron-deficiency anemia, hardening of the arteries, infertility, skin disorders and other diseases, emphasize the importance of trace elements in human health. Zinc has also been shown to be an important ingredient in healing wounds, especially burns, and in the repair of bones and arteries. Its balance in the body is a known essential in the metabolism of two amino acids and in the activity of several enzyme systems."

The university researchers believe that facts like these can lead to important, perhaps life-saving findings for human beings. One test turned up evidence that the more phosphorus farmers apply to their soil, the less zinc there may be in corn grown there. Phosphorus, as we stated, is one of the main ingredients of most commercial fertilizers. Zinc is not. This is one way we produce trace mineral imbalances in food.

"Results of this nature suggest that one should examine carefully the long-term effects of heavy fertilization rated from the standpoint of human health," said Dr. Singh. "However, man doesn't live by sweet corn alone, and such deficiencies can be easily corrected by other foods. Whether all crops show this phosphorus-zinc antagonism hasn't been determined. If they do, this could lead to serious nutritional deficiencies in under-developed rural areas where most of the food is secured from one type of soil."

These West Virginia findings point up the importance of a recent test which found that, in 11 Midwestern states, the iron, copper, zinc and manganese content of grain has dropped *in the last four years.*

"Changes in the nutrient composition of plants could have far-reaching effects on the health of animals and the men that consume them," Dr. Singh said. "The importance of trace elements in human nutrition is obvious, and more research in this area should be carried out. Our study on sweet corn is offered as a model only because a single dietary ingredient in man's nutritional status isn't likely to be significant."

Dr. Henry Schroeder says that about 7,000 tons of copper are sprayed on vines, trees and other crops every year in the United States. This is not toxic, he reports. About 25,000 tons of yellow sulfur are dusted every year as fungicides. It hurts no one, according to Dr. Schroeder. Other trace minerals used in agricultural applications are barium, boron, selenium, antimony and thallium. Lead arsenate is sometimes used as a pesticide. "So much lead, copper, sodium and calcium arsenates have been added to some soils that crops, including fruits, will contain arsenic for many years. Tobacco is frequently sprayed with arsenic, and some people have suggested that lung cancer in smokers comes from the arsenic," Dr. Schroeder says.

A startling new approach to the need for farming with compost and the potential contamination of waterways with fluoride from commercial fertilizers is presented in the April-May, 1972 issue of *Compost Science*. It seems that most of the commercial fertilizers like superphosphate and rock phosphate contain lots of fluorine, which leaches out into soil and hence into waterways. Lake Erie is already threatened with "death"—that is, eutrophication caused partly by the phosphates and nitrates used in commercial fertilizers which wash into the lake.

Albert Schatz and Vivian Schatz of Temple University and Radburn Research Institute write that the nitrate in fertilizers is also responsible for bringing about contamination of drinking water in many places, so that children who drink the water suffer from a possibly fatal blood disorder, methemoglobinemia. Adults who get too much nitrate in their food also risk cancer, since this substance reacts with other chemicals in food to produce a substance which is known to cause cancer.

As for fluorine, using 1,000 pounds of superphosphate on an acre of soil adds about 17½ pounds of fluorine. It's a contaminant of the fertilizer. This increases the fluorine content of the soil to about 7½ ppm. Drs. Schatz give us several references to studies which show that plants pick up fluorine from soil. In 1946, a USDA study showed that fluorine accumulated in every one of four New Jersey soils fertilized with superphosphate.

Several years earlier, University of Wisconsin scientists found that relatively large amounts of fluorine escape into drainage water from both kinds of phosphate fertilizer. In one case the drainage water contained 1.7 ppm of fluorine, which approaches the 2 ppm level which produces tooth mottling. Under some circumstances, the drainage water might contain as much as 6.3 ppm of fluorine. The Wisconsin scientists concluded that "when phosphate fertilization is carried on over many years, very considerable quantities of highly toxic fluorine will have been added to the soil." Two USDA scientists, studying the amount of fluorine in plants grown on fields which had been fertilized with superphosphate for 15 years, found that spinach plants contained 28.3 ppm and poke shoots contained 42.3 ppm of fluorine.

Japanese investigators also found alarming increases in fluorine content of foods grown in heavily fertilized soil. The fluorine content of some foods rose by as much as 967 per cent! Because of this the daily average consumption of fluorine in food in that locality rose from 3.21 mg. to 8.82 mg. per day—an increase of 175 per cent.

The two Japanese scientists collected statistics on cancer deaths and found that there were more deaths from stomach cancer in areas where rice had a high fluorine content. There were also more such deaths in areas where large amounts of phosphate fertilizers had been used.

As recently as 1970 Russian scientists have voiced concern over a possibility of fluorine causing cancer. In 1965, University of Texas researchers found that fluorine in drinking water accelerated the growth of tumor transplants in mice and embryonated eggs. Other references are given in the Schatz article for further evidence that fluorine may cause cancer.

The Schatz team presents compelling evidence that compost used instead of phosphate fertilizers will solve the problem. The organic, living things in garbage and other wastes which are used to make compost do not contain the fluorine which is inherent in phosphate fertilizers.

Almost everyone agrees that we should be returning to the soil all wastes that can be broken down into soil components, without damage from contaminants. Even the defenders of commercial fertilizers parrot the environmentalist's cry to recycle everything that can be recycled. Of course, they say, we should be composting garbage

CHAPTER 29

Are You Absorbing the Minerals From Your Diet?

LET'S SAY YOU have designed for yourself the best possible diet. You've checked carefully to include enough of each of the important groups of foods—the high-protein meat, fish, poultry, eggs and dairy products; the high-protein seed foods including wholegrain cereals, wheat germ and bran, as well as nuts, beans, soybeans, peas and seeds like sunflower seeds; the vegetables, especially the dark green leafy ones, so rich in B vitamins, vitamin A, C and many minerals, and the fruits which give you vitamin C, vitamin A and potassium in abundance.

You've cut out all the unnecessary foods that would otherwise dilute your meals—the ones that contribute nothing but empty calories in the way of sugars and fats. Now can you settle back, secure in the knowledge there's not one more thing you can do to guarantee good nutrition?

Not quite. There's still the question of absorption. Are you certain you will absorb all the nutrients you need from such a good diet? There are hazards. Some people suffer from diseases which make it impossible to absorb much of what they eat. Chronic diarrhea and dysentery bring about the loss of much valuable nutrient as well as water. Celiac disease and related conditions in which the cereal protein gluten causes trouble bring about losses of nutrients until a diet which excludes gluten is used.

Another hazard is just getting old. Yes, it seems that, along with all the other disadvantages of growing older, we must contend with reduced ability to absorb as much of the nutrients in our daily meals as we could absorb when we were younger.

Dr. William H. Strain, whom we quoted earlier when he was at the University of Rochester, and who is now at the University of Missouri, recently presented a paper at the 10th Annual Conference on Trace Minerals in Environmental Health. In it he described experiments he and his associates did with radioactive tracers of iron and zinc to determine the amount absorbed by animals of different sexes and ages. By a process called "whole-body counting," the scientists could locate each particle of the dose of iron or zinc they had given the animal, hence discover how much was absorbed and how much had been excreted.

Anemia is the disease of iron deficiency, as we know. There is a disease of zinc deficiency called *acrodermatitis enteropathica* or AE. It's rare but very disabling and, in the past, usually fatal. Now doctors have discovered they can treat it by giving the trace mineral zinc. Laboratory scientists have measured the amount of zinc in the bodies of patients with AE and compared it to the amount of zinc in the bodies of well volunteers. In every case the AE patient absorbed only about one-fourth of the zinc he was given. The normal person absorbs about two-thirds of the zinc given.

Scientists are trying to discover how and why this happens. It is not easy. Dr. Strain says, "The mechanism of intestinal absorption has been and will continue to be a major problem of mineral metabolism." Doctors know that getting too much iron can be serious, perhaps fatal, to very young children. There are reports in medical literature of children who have eaten a whole bottle of iron pills and become very ill. The reason the iron acts so drastically is not known, says Dr. Strain.

It is known that deficiencies of minerals occur most frequently in older folks, presumably because their intestines just do not absorb the minerals as they did when these people were young. "There are many gaps in understanding the changes with age in the absorption and metabolism of iron, zinc and other minerals," says Dr. Strain.

Dr. Strain fed measured amounts of zinc and iron to his laboratory rats, then measured the amount of each mineral left in the body of the animal. His study showed that both iron and zinc were retained and absorbed more by young than by old rats and larger amounts were absorbed by females than by male rats. In younger animals this sex effect was not very pronounced. But in year-old animals it was obvious that the females retained more. And, interestingly enough, older female rats which had had many offspring retained more of the minerals than young, virgin female rats.

This seems to demonstrate nature's provision for the young. Young females and even older females which are breeding need more minerals to provide strength and growth for their offspring. Once retired from the breeding program, the female rats began to absorb less of the minerals.

Iron is the trace mineral which carries oxygen in the blood to all body cells. Without enough of it, weakness and easy fatigue, susceptibility to infections, lassitude and poor mental functioning will result. A recent survey showed that about 15 percent of all Americans examined were short on iron. There is no reason for this except unwise selection of food and neglect of food supplements.

Still another hazard is immobilization due to illness. If you have visited a rest home or nursing home, you have probably been appalled at the number of older people who appear to be completely immobilized. Although conscious and not suffering from any acute disorder, they lie in bed constantly or they sit in wheel chairs from which they are apparently never moved, except to return to bed.

MINERALS: KILL OR CURE?

An important study of this situation was reported in the August, 1975 issue of the *Journal of the American Geriatrics Society*. Michael B. Miller, M.D., FACP, discusses the eventual effects of such immobility on nursing home patients. They are horrible to contemplate. And they can be reversed by special therapy. There is no need for prolonged inactivity of most patients. And their immobilization makes more work for the nursing staff and doctors, as well as more expense for everyone concerned. Dr. Miller calls these sad effects of immobilization "iatrogenic" (which means caused by doctors) or "nurisgenic" (caused by nurses.)

He tells us first of the great importance of two things in preventing harm to bones—first the mineral calcium in ample amounts every day. There is no indication that our needs for calcium decrease as we age. Indeed, they seem to increase. In women past menopause one early symptom of osteoporosis (or soft bones) is what is known as "dowagers hump"—a not very attractive hump at the back of the neck. Next time you are in church or at a concert, observe the back of the necks of the women sitting in front of you and estimate how many of them are getting too little calcium at meals.

The second most important element in this quite serious disorder which affects older people who are immobilized is the lack of what doctors call "skeletal stress." It seems that bones, to be healthy, must be in constant use. This is especially true of those which bear weight—the pelvis, hip bones and leg bones. They were designed by nature to bear weight. As soon as this weight is removed and the individual lies motionless in bed or sits in a wheel chair, those bones begin to disintegrate. If there is an accompanying lack of calcium, osteoporosis is almost certain. Osteoporosis, as we discuss in more detail beginning on page 63, is the softening of bones, as minerals are withdrawn and the bones become unable to bear weight.

Calcium, phosphorus, potassium and other minerals are lost in urine and feces when one is immobile. This makes the situation worse. It is well known that circulatory troubles also increase during bed rest, for the simple reason that the valves in the legs do not function properly unless one is up and about. Walking purposefully and briskly is the best way to keep these valves pumping blood along the blood vessels in the leg so that it does not accumulate, become sluggish and clot. The additional loss of so many minerals from bones compounds the health problems.

But, as Dr. Miller tells us, prolonged immobilization affects the personality and the social outlook of the bedridden person. He gives us case reports of six elderly women who were put to bed in a nursing home because of broken hips, heart disorders, infections, amputations and so on. After four weeks of immobilization, they had apparently decided they were dying and they began to behave appropriately. They stopped eating and drinking fluids. They stopped talking. They refused to communicate in any way with nurses or doctors.

If nurses tried to feed them, they spit out the food. Several of them became incontinent of urine and feces. If they were placed in wheelchairs they deliberately caused accidents. When nurses attempted to get them to stand, they went through a series of bizarre movements all calculated to prevent themselves from standing. If they were helped up, their knees collapsed beneath them and they fell to the floor.

Throughout all this there was no measurable evidence of any damage to legs or nerves. True, muscles had wasted and bones were deteriorating because of the prolonged bedrest, but the personality changes, too, appeared to have no other basis except the fact that they had been confined to bed for so long.

Says Dr. Miller, "the syndrome is reversible." These old folks can be gotten on their feet. They can be rehabilitated. They can learn to feed themselves once again. They will once again begin to communicate with those around them and become part of the social life of the establishment. After their rehabilitation they will admit that they thought they were dying and resigned themselves to it. The only reason for this conviction was the total effect upon them of prolonged immobilization.

Dr. Miller says, "In the absence of continuing and direct medical involvement in the progressive rehabilitation of the severely disabled aged patient in whom total disability is exacerbated by the onset of acute illness, the nursing staff in a long-term care facility must assume responsibility for nursing rehabilitation even when such maneuvers require the removal of restraints ordered by physicians. Responsibility for the safety of the patient thus accrues to the nursing staff....Iatrogenic factors in producing the patient's disability have long been recognized. Nurisgenic factors are now coming to the fore."

In other words, doctors in general are not aware of the damage being done to their long-term patients who are immobilized. Or, if they are, they seem not to know what to do about it. So it is the job of the nurses who are with these patients all day to get them out of bed and out of wheelchairs for their own salvation. Of course, as they become, once again, able to care for themselves, to bathe, clothe and feed themselves, the work of the nurses is greatly decreased.

The reason for the original immobilization, which brings all these terrible consequences is, usually, breaking a bone, having a heart attack or some other circulatory disorder or related disease which disables the older person. So the sensible person will do everything possible to avoid such health disasters. For, at any age, prolonged immobilization will bring serious side effects.

The broken bones which accompany falls in older people are usually not caused by the fall; the bone just disintegrates and becomes so fragile that it cannot support weight. So it collapses and the individual falls. Plenty of minerals in the diet—chiefly calcium—is the only way to prevent these emergencies.

It helps to have some fat in your digestive tract at the same time as the calcium, so you probably absorb more calcium from whole milk than from skim milk. On the other hand too much fat causes you to lose calcium. As always, be moderate.

Vitamin D is essential for the absorption of calcium. You get vitamin D from sunlight in summer and spring, if you are outside part of the day. In winter, especially in northern states, it's a good idea to take some vitamin D—every week or so, since it is fat-soluble and your body retains it well.

Recently, health food stores have begun to sell chelated minerals, which are discussed in more detail in another chapter. This is a form of the mineral which is easier to absorb than other forms. Chelating agents have been used for many years in animal feed to guarantee that the minerals in the feed are fully absorbed by the animals. There are natural chelates as well. Casein—a protein in milk—and liver extract contain chelates which make it possible for anyone eating milk products or liver to absorb more zinc, for example. Natural and synthetic chelates are used in chick feed so that the young animals make better use of the zinc in the soybean mixtures they are fed.

As usual, preparations which are known to be helpful to plants and animals come only belatedly to human beings. Because there is no cash value to human beings, we don't usually get the professional care which profitable plant and animal crops get. But now chelated minerals are available for us. You can try them and see if your absorption of various minerals improves.

How can you tell? Your health should improve—not immediately, but eventually. If you have been short on iron the improvement may be quite rapid if you take chelated iron. And, incidentally, diets high in fiber—and we hope that's the kind you're eating—tend to entail bulky stools in which some body iron may be lost. So taking this mineral will help to keep you in balance.

CHAPTER 30

What Are Chelated Minerals?

"IRON DEFICIENCY IS a nutritional problem of world-wide medical concern," say four researchers in the *American Journal of Clinical Nutrition* for October, 1972. "The prevalence of anemias in this country is an embarrassing reminder that iron fortification of various foods like bread might be improved with respect to the assimilability of the iron supplement."

Ever since iron deficiency anemia was diagnosed by physicians, getting enough iron into the anemic person in the proper form for absorption has been a major problem. The ancients tried to solve it by soaking iron until it became rusty, then giving the patient the rusty water to drink. No doubt some small amount of this iron was retained and gave some relief.

In modern times, various forms of iron have been used in medicines and food supplements, without very much success in getting the mineral to stay where it belongs in the body, rather than just being excreted. By giving huge doses doctors hope to get absorption of at least some iron. But many iron preparations may cause unpleasant side effects—abdominal discomfort and/or diarrhea, for example. When anemic patients cannot stand the side effects, iron preparations are sometimes injected.

Although iron deficiency anemia is apparently widespread in our country—in spite of the "enrichment" of white bread with iron—it seems likely that absorption of other minerals may be just as chancy as that of iron. How do we know, for example, how many people have efficient body mechanisms for absorbing all the chromium from their food, or the copper or the potassium? Mightn't it be a good idea to give the essential minerals and trace minerals in a form that assures good absorption, just to be certain we are making progress in preventing nationwide shortages of these nutrients, in these days when mineral-deficient processed foods make up such a large part of American meals?

Dr. George W. Bates and his colleagues report in the *American Journal of Clinical Nutrition* on their experiment giving iron in the form of ferric fructose. They tested guinea pigs with this form of iron, tracing the amount of the mineral that remained in the blood cells. And they tested the same guinea pigs using iron sulfate, which is the form in which iron is most usually given by doctors to anemic people.

During the first day after the supplement was given, *60 percent of both preparations was excreted*. During the next two days the rate of excretion declined. At the end of two weeks, no iron was being excreted and the percentage of iron absorbed from the ferric fructose *was three times that from the sulfate preparation*.

Ferric fructose is "chelated" iron. This means that the way in which the iron is bound chemically to the fructose helps the intestine to absorb the iron. Thus, when we speak of chelated minerals, we mean that they have been treated or "chelated" so that they are more readily absorbed. The authors of this article say they believe this evidence of availability of chelated iron gives hope for enriching many foods with such a product. They suggest using it in soft drinks, candy, cakes and other foods, especially those most popular with children.

So far as we know, nothing has been done about this suggestion. Most of us are still getting little absorbable iron and other minerals if we eat white sugar and white flour, white bread and processed cereals as well as desserts.

There has been one great step forward in the effort to offer not just iron but all essential minerals in a form that is easily absorbed. Not surprisingly, these products are available first in health food stores. Somehow you always find there the most nourishing products which the giant food industry and the drug industry haven't yet discovered. Chelated minerals are now available to all of us.

These minerals are chelated with amino acids or forms of protein, as the iron was chelated with fructose in the experiment described above. In the Summer, 1976 issue of the *Journal of Applied Nutrition*, M. Taher Fouad, M.Sc., Ph.D., describes the way in which the body (and scientists) discriminate between essential and non-essential minerals. An essential mineral is one which is present in all healthy tissues of all living things. Its concentration in these is relatively constant. Lack of this mineral in these tissues produces abnormalities which are reversed or prevented by giving the mineral in a form that can be absorbed. If a mineral is in the body only as a result of contamination of food or environment (as is the case with toxic lead and cadmium), such minerals are known not to be essential, but to be harmful instead.

The body has a chemical mechanism whereby it controls its levels of minerals, restores the correct concentrations and brings about a normal distribution of minerals and trace minerals in all tissues. But in the case of the non-essential, toxic ones, there often is no such mechanism, hence the toxicity.

As we have indicated in this book, essential trace minerals are: chromium, cobalt, copper, fluorine, iron, iodine, manganese, molybdenum, nickel, selenium, silicon, tin, vanadium and zinc. Says Dr. Fouad, "Only within the past five years fluoride, nickel, tin, selenium, silicon and vanadium have been added to the group of essential trace elements. Although these essential trace elements are completely indispensable to cellular and body biological functions, yet, if they enter the cell or organism in large amounts, they become toxic...increasing amounts of certain elements result in stimulating biological response until a plateau is reached. If intakes exceed this amount, a (drug) action followed by toxic effects will appear. Thus fluorine and selenium, which were long considered to be poisons, are now identified as essential nutrients, since their metabolic role is essential to specific biological functions." But in large doses they are toxic.

The first necessity for proper absorption of trace minerals is a healthy, normal digestive tract, says Dr. Fouad, especially in that part of the intestine where mineral absorption takes place. In cases of diarrhea (and many Americans suffer from chronic diarrheal states), potassium may not be absorbed and profound weakness of muscles may follow. Chelation of the trace minerals helps the digestive system of the body to absorb the mineral—even the disordered digestive system. But the mineral must be in a chelated form. For instance, the trace mineral cobalt is not absorbed except as it occurs as an integral part of vitamin B12.

It's true, too, that imbalances in the various trace minerals can create imbalances in the body. Too much iron medication can cause deficiency in copper, although a certain small amount of copper is essential for iron absorption. Too much calcium has been found to create iron deficiency in one group of children and iron and zinc deficiency in another group. Zinc depresses the body's ability to absorb copper and vice versa. So chelated minerals must be used with care so as to avoid imbalances.

This is why they are so carefully formulated, with, in every instance, the Recommended Dietary Allowance in mind; or, in the case of those minerals for which there is no RDA, the amounts suggested by experts in the field as the optimal amounts. In addition to these safeguards, common sense should be your guide.

Obviously, if your drinking water has been fluoridated for

many years, you should not consider taking chelated fluoride. If you take vitamin B12 shots or a sizable vitamin B12 pill frequently, you undoubtedly don't need chelated cobalt, which is already in this vitamin B12. On the other hand, if you have eaten white bread and lots of white sugar most of your life, chances are very good that some additional zinc, magnesium and manganese would be helpful, since you have probably suffered from a more or less deficient state in these three trace minerals for many years. A chelated source of these three minerals might prove very valuable.

In one experiment involving human subjects, those who suffered from gout reported that they found relief from their gouty symptoms when they took chelated magnesium. In the same experiment, reported by Ned L. Jensen, hair analyses showed optimal increases in trace minerals. It is customary to test hair samples to detect the amount of the trace minerals present in the body. Some interesting things developed with the trace mineral zinc in this test which seemed to indicate that sex hormones have considerable influence over the absorption of zinc. The men volunteers had only slight increases in the zinc in their hair, although they had considerably more zinc in their blood. In the women, zinc increased greatly in the hair, and iron and copper decreased. Zinc is thought to be essential for the health of the prostate gland and other male organs of reproduction and possibly very helpful in preventing disorders in this area. Prostate disorders are unknown in parts of the world where traditional diets are eaten and processed foods are unknown. Does this not suggest that deficiency in B vitamins and trace minerals may be at least partly responsible for our nationwide plague of prostate disorders?

All the subjects, male and female, got the same amount of chelated iron and apparently absorbed about the same amount. The average hemoglobin (the blood element by which anemia is measured) went up approximately two milligrams percent during the experiment, indicating that the chelated iron was well absorbed.

Dr. Fouad tell us that iron is absorbed better from meals in which there is some good source of natural iron like meat, fish or poultry, while meals in which the protein is supplied by milk products (low in iron) did not encourage the absorption of iron. In the case of manganese, a diabetic patient did not respond to insulin with a lowered blood sugar level until manganese was added, when the situation righted itself, seeming to indicate that this mineral is especially essential for those with disordered blood sugar levels. In another study, a natural diet high in manganese was replaced with a commercial diet. The laboratory animal being studied became diabetic. Giving insulin was not effective. But restoring the original amount of manganese to the diet brought blood sugar levels back to normal.

The amount of selenium in blood may be 10-fold higher in areas where there are comparatively high levels of selenium in food and water, whereas in those areas where this trace mineral is lacking, blood levels will reflect this lack. A number of body enzymes depend for their effectiveness on selenium. In an experiment with rabbits, giving the trace mineral vanadium helped to decrease cholesterol levels in blood. The same was later confirmed in experiments with human beings.

In the case of zinc, Dr. Fouad tells us that zinc compounded with two amino acids or forms or protein (chelated zinc) was found in the blood within 15 minutes after the tablet was taken. Maximum amounts of zinc were found in the blood after four hours. The following body organs later showed rapid uptake of zinc from the chelated mineral tablet, seeming to indicate that this trace mineral is an essential element in the health of these organs: liver, kidney, spleen, intestinal lining, lung, pancreas, thyroid, pituitary, testes and adrenals.

According to William W. Seroy, writing in Vol. 1, No. 6 of *World Health and Ecology News*, May, 1971, we miss out on much of our mineral intake. That is, we just don't absorb all the minerals that we eat, for one reason or another. Mr. Seroy tells us that, 15 years ago, three biologists became concerned over what was happening to trace minerals in the soil and in the animals that eat food grown there.

"First," he says, "they set about to find out why inorganic (metallic) trace minerals were not as readily assimilated by the body as were organic minerals. Their research carried them all the way from studying trace mineral levels in the soils and comparing this to the levels in foodstuffs grown in this soil to the transportation and evolvement of trace minerals in actual living tissue.

"Absorption is no doubt a major problem in considering the nourishment of the human body," he went on. "All food factors reaching the upper intestinal tract are not absorbed uniformly and adequately. In order to explain this we must compare the body to an automobile battery and its electromotive potential. The animal body may be thought of as a very complex battery that not only receives, stores and uses electrical energy for chemical purposes, but also maintains itself by assimilating the vitamins, minerals, amino acids, and other nutrients needed to meet its daily functions."

Food contains both negative and positive charged particles called ions. The negatively charged particles pass through the intestinal wall quite easily. But the positively charged particles do not pass through so easily, hence are mostly lost to the body, since they pass out through the bowel in feces.

As a result, according to this article, four-fifths of the organic trace minerals are lost and only one-fifth gets through to the cells to be used in the many activities in which these minerals participate.

For example, only one milligram in every 10 milligrams of iron that we eat is absorbed by the intestines into the blood and used by the body. The rest is lost. It seems wasteful, does it not?

Several years ago, the three biologists referred to above—Harvey G. Ashmead, Ph.D., Phil Hinze, DVM, and Darrel Graff, Ph.D.—began to experiment with several of these trace minerals—iron, zinc, copper and cobalt—to see if they might be able to obtain a greater rate of absorption. They found that by chelating or complexing these minerals with amino acids they could increase the assimilation of the mineral into the body sometimes as much as 300 percent. They measured this by analyzing the hair, feathers and tissue of the animals and birds who were fed the chelated minerals.

Mr. Seroy tells us that "the process of chelation (pronounced key-layshun) is the means of surrounding or enclosing a mineral atom by a larger protein molecule." He then describes the chemical process by which this is done. The result is that the minerals can be transported readily through intestinal walls, into the blood and thence into the cells where they are most needed.

The process, in essence, changes an inorganic mineral into an organic one. So the problem of absorption or assimilation has been overcome, and we now have available a whole new field of mineral therapy never before known.

Here, for example, is the result of a study using laboratory rats. The scientists chelated four minerals—copper, magnesium, iron and zinc. They gave them to the animals along with their usual chow. They kept one group of rats as "controls" which got no chelated minerals.

The rats taking the chelated supplements absorbed the following amounts of the minerals:

Copper......................33 parts per million (ppm)
Magnesium ....94 parts per million
Iron....................................298 parts per million
Zinc....................................191 parts per million

Those rats which got no supplements at all were found to have absorbed from their food only a trace of copper, 7 ppm of magnesium, 23 ppm of iron and 14 ppm of zinc.

Animals taking only *inorganic* forms of the minerals absorbed them as follows: 12 ppm and 8 ppm of copper, 77 ppm and 36 ppm of magnesium, 171 and 78 ppm of iron, and 87 and 84 ppm of zinc. It is obvious that the chelated form of all these minerals was far superior to the inorganic forms in terms of the amount of mineral absorbed.

Farmers and gardeners know that chelated minerals are taken up much more readily and quickly by plants, producing superior crops laden with trace minerals. Corn was found in one experiment to germinate quicker and grow higher when chelated minerals were added to the soil.

Poultrymen have found that chelated minerals given in feed increase egg laying, produce better quality feathers, protect the poultry from disease, produce harder egg shells and tougher shell membranes.

In raising pigs, a very common condition of anemia among litters has been prevented by giving the mothers chelated iron during pregnancy. Weight gain among the piglets has been 2.65 pounds more per piglet than among those animals whose mothers did not get the chelated mineral.

In fish hatcheries, fingerlings grow much faster. A weakness in leg muscles in turkeys is prevented by chelated minerals. Sperm count in bulls is increased, greatly increasing breeding efficiency.

In all, says Mr. Seroy, over 200,000 animals have been given chelated minerals experimentally. In almost every case mineral levels in their bodies were favorably increased. The beneficial effects were noted in better growth in the young and better production.

No toxicity has been reported—another great advantage of chelated minerals over inorganic ones. Aside from being much better absorbed, so that minerals are not simply wasted by being excreted, the chelated ones are much safer if taken in quantity.

What about human beings? One study involved 65 volunteers divided into 10 control groups. The first took a supplement of assorted chelated minerals. The second group took the same minerals plus a one-a-day vitamin tablet. Group 3 took 1.2 grams of chelated calcium with vitamins. Group 4 took 75 milligrams of chelated magnesium with vitamins. Group 5 took 75 milligrams of chelated zinc with vitamins. Group 6 took 75 milligrams of chelated iron with vitamins.

Group 7 took 30 milligrams of chelated manganese with vitamins. Group 8 took 10 milligrams of chelated copper with vitamins, and Group 9 took 1.3 grams of chelated phosphorus with vitamins. The tenth group took only vitamins. The scientists took samples of hair, urine, saliva and blood to test before and after supplementation.

In the first group, general health seemed improved and minerals in the hair samples were more balanced. In the second group there was also improvement in health. In the third group, there were large increases of calcium in the hair sample. "Chelated calcium is very actively absorbed and should be dealt with carefully," says the report.

In Group 4, there were increased amounts of both calcium and magnesium in the hair sample. Some of the volunteers found that their gout had improved apparently from the extra magnesium.

In Group 5 an interesting difference in sex was observed. In the women volunteers the zinc level of the hair increased greatly and the iron and copper level decreased. In the men, the opposite was the case. Volunteers in this group reported increasing fatigue as the experiment proceeded. "The daily dose of 75 milligrams is perhaps too high for extended periods," say the authors.

In Group 6 all participants felt better and showed no side effects. The average hemoglobin count went up approximately two milligrams percent.

In Group 7, chelated manganese increased in the hair and increased slightly in the blood. Volunteers reported better health, no side effects.

In Group 8, the copper supplement of five times the official recommended allowance caused some mild toxicity in the form of intestinal cramps, nerve sensitivity and diarrhea after three weeks. Small pains that do not generally bother people became annoying. These volunteers also had a loss of calcium in the hair. Apparently copper is antagonistic to calcium.

The group taking the chelated phosphorus reported strong

diuretic action—that is, increased urine in which large amounts of potassium, magnesium and calcium were lost. All these volunteers experienced cramps and side effects.

In general, say the authors, chelated minerals are absorbed better than inorganic ones. Copper and phosphorus may be toxic when given singly. Vitamins seem to help balance minerals in the body. And it seems a good idea to take balanced minerals, especially if you are taking the chelated ones. Taking larger than usual amounts of just one or two may unbalance some of the others.

With the ever-increasing pollution of our environment with chemical poisons, public health officials are understandably concerned with ways to remove toxic trace minerals from the bodies of people who have been exposed to excessive doses. City children who have far too much lead in their bodies for good health, for example, should not simply be left to suffer from lead poisoning.

Fortunately, there is a group of compounds which, when used by experienced physicians, can remove some of these toxic materials from the body harmlessly. A substance with the ominous sounding name of *ethylenediamine-tetraacetic acid* (EDTA for short) can be given to people suffering from poisoning from some metal and the drug will combine with the metal in a chelating action and cause it to be excreted harmlessly. Basically, the chelate "ties up" or binds the metal, so that it becomes unavailable to the body. Then it is safely excreted. EDTA forms compounds that are very stable—they hold the metal tightly until it is disposed of.

Here are the names of some chelating agents and the metals which they chelate or render harmless:

EDTA can be used against cadmium, chromium, cobalt, copper, lead, manganese, nickel, radium, selenium, tungsten, uranium, vanadium and zinc.

Dimercaprol, another chelating agent, is used by doctors to detoxify people who have, in one way or another, gotten too much of these metals in their bodies: antimony, arsenic, bismuth, gold, lead (it is used with EDTA to chelate lead), mercury, nickel and tungsten.

Anyone who gets too much iron can be treated with a drug called *deferoxamine*, which chelates the iron and gets rid of it innocuously.

Thallium is a poison used in rat, ant and roach poisons. Someone who accidentally ingests such a poison may be given by his doctor a chelating agent called *Dithiocarb* or one called *Dithizon*. This information is from the classic physician's reference book, *The Merck Manual*, 12th Edition.

A certain disease called "polycythemia" involves the making of too many red blood cells in the body. Too much cobalt can induce this disease in rats, mice, guinea pigs, dogs, pigs, ducks, chickens and human beings. EDTA given along with cobalt apparently ties up the cobalt in a chelating action and the disease does not appear. One might think it is unlikely that most of us will ever have to use this knowledge, since cobalt has a fairly low order of toxicity and we are not exposed, generally speaking, to large amounts of it. But, as we related in an earlier chapter, there was a recent incident in which a number of heavy drinkers—drinking beer contaminated with cobalt—suffered severe heart damage. EDTA was given to remove the cobalt from their bodies. And EDTA, incidentally, is used to make iron in soil more available to plants. Chelates of iron can be put into the soil or sprayed on the plants.

As we have mentioned, chelated minerals can be used in animal feed to increase the animals' absorption of various minerals. Dr. E. J. Underwood tells us that certain natural feeds contain natural chelating substances. Casein (a protein in milk) and liver extract contain chelates which improve the absorption and utilization of zinc. Several natural and synthetic chelating agents in their food improve the availability of zinc to chicks which are eating mostly protein from soybeans.

As scientists devote more time to the study of trace minerals and the efficiency of chelated minerals where absorption is concerned, much more information will become available on this subject. Meanwhile, there seems to be no reason not to take advantage of those products which are available. Use your common sense in taking chelated minerals. First, check with your doctor or have a hair analysis made, if possible, to see which minerals may be lacking or present in insufficient amounts. And it's probably best to take an all-in-one mineral supplement where the comparative amounts of these elements are carefully balanced, so that you will not get too much of one, too little of another. Since the chelated minerals are so well absorbed, there is no need to take more than you may need. If, after the hair analysis, your doctor determines that you need more of a specific mineral, this mineral is probably available in chelated form at your health food store.

If you wish to have the mineral content of your hair analyzed, there are several places where this can be done. One of these is The Life-Extension & Control of Ageing Program, 2223 L Street, Sacramento, California 95802. Details are available in some 900 health food stores in the United States, or you can write directly to the Mineral Evaluation by Hair Analysis at the above address.

CHAPTER 31

More on Minerals

JENIFER JOWSEY, PH.D., director of orthopedic research at the Mayo Clinic, Rochester, Minnesota, told an audience at the Sixth Annual California Dairy Council meeting in 1976 that the average American diet, high in phosphorus and low in calcium almost guarantees osteoporosis in later life.

Osteoporosis, as we learned in an earlier chapter, is the disease in which bones become soft and brittle, causing a general shrinkage of the skeleton, a "dowager's hump" at the back of the neck, pain in the lower back and, in some cases, malfunction of the lungs. It is especially common among women after menopause. Part of the reason is just plain lack of the mineral calcium at meals. Part of the reason is the prevalence of diets high in phosphorus which disrupt the important balance between these two minerals.

Said Dr. Jowsey, "Americans in general tend to decrease their intake of calcium as they get older. However, the shift from big meals to snack foods has caused phosphorus intake to go up and calcium intake to go down in the United States." Foods which contain a great deal of phosphorus and little calcium are: fish, poultry, meat, cereals and bread. Dairy products, too, are rich in phosphorus, although they are also our best source of calcium.

All these are fine foods—no reason to slight them. But, says Dr. Jowsey, if you want to avoid the painful and disfiguring disease of osteoporosis in later life, you must somehow manage to get more calcium. She suggests taking calcium supplements, not just after middleage when you become concerned about the dangers of softened, brittle bones, but from the age of 25 on. Take supplemental calcium up to one gram daily in the form of calcium tablets, she says, if you want to avoid osteoporosis in later life. If you haven't done this earlier in life, of course, the next best thing is to begin now to use calcium supplements daily.

The official recommendation of calcium intake is 800 milligrams a day for adults. Dr. Jowsey believes we need more than that and a number of prominent researchers in this field agree with her. They, too, suggest 1,000 milligrams daily in a supplement—that is, in addition to the amount in food.

Dr. Jowsey says it is essential for life that the level of calcium in the blood remains normal. "When there is an abnormal absorption of this element in the stomach and intestines or when too much calcium is lost in the kidney, the skeleton provides the only source of calcium. Bone tissue is resorbed (taken away, borrowed) to put more calcium in the blood." The same thing happens when the diet is too high in phosphorus without enough calcium to balance it.

"If you want to end up at 70 with the skeleton of a 16-year-old, start supplementing your diet with calcium at age 25," says Dr. Jowsey.

She mentions two other aspects of life which are related to the way our bodies use calcium. Alcoholic drinks tend to make us lose calcium. Half of all the calcium we get in food may be lost if we drink something alcoholic at the same time. The other important thing to keep in mind is activity. Daily activity is absolutely essential to keep bones healthy. Inactivity (very common in older women) prevents stress to the bones. And they need stress—the stress of holding the body upright, of supporting the legs, hips and arms during strenuous activity. Just going for a 15-minute walk or taking 20 minutes of exercise is not enough, says Dr. Jowsey. "One needs to be active throughout the day for the proper stress effects to occur."

Dr. Jowsey did not mention it, but it is well to keep in

mind, also, that other food elements are essential to one's absorption of calcium. Vitamin D must be present for calcium to be absorbed properly. It helps if lactose is also present. This is milk sugar. So taking your calcium tablets with some milk will help the absorption. Either too much or too little fat in the intestines at the same time you take calcium tends to prevent absorption. This is one reason for avoiding diets which sharply restrict fat. It is also a good reason for not living on diets extremely high in fat.

Some recent investigation seemed to show that taking calcium supplements at bedtime is preferable to taking them during the day. A number of women with osteoporosis who took their calcium supplements just before going to bed retained considerably more calcium than those who took them during the day.

A University of Rochester scientist has discovered, he says, that calcium in the diet reduces tooth decay. He could, of course, have discovered this fact by reading some of the health food literature of the past 50 years or so. But, no. He fed animals tooth-decay-causing foods—chiefly snacks and commercial cereals loaded with sugar. And he produced rampant tooth decay in the animals.

Then he added calcium lactate to the sugar-laden foods and produced a 50 percent reduction in tooth decay. The doctor says there are no known bad effects connected with "the drug" as scientists prefer to call nutrients when they give them to prevent some illness.

Why, said the scientist, we could add this calcium to all the sugar-laden foods without destroying the taste of them and thus could cut in half the incidence of tooth decay in children. Just what the health food movement has said for many years when they recommended bone meal, dolomite, calcium lactate or any other calcium preparation to prevent tooth decay.

Of course, at the same time we do not recommend the sugar-containing snacks and cereals. It seems never to occur to a scientist working in the field of tooth health that something which is destructive to teeth is also probably equally destructive to other parts of the body. As is becoming increasingly evident these days, eating sugar in the amounts in which we eat it is the single most destructive eating habit we have.

A recent veterinarian's column printed a letter from a reader who said, "My husband considers me a food faddist. I know what is good for me and try to eat it. One of our disagreements concerns milk versus yogurt. I consider the latter vastly superior to milk. I whip up this yogurt drink which I know is better for me and it's even better for our dog, Dixie. She can drink the yogurt and does famously on it. Whenever she drinks that much milk, she gets diarrhea. I feel that's further proof of yogurt's superiority as a natural food. Do you agree?"

The vet answered as follows: "Dixie's diarrhea brought on by milk consumption is probably related to the lactose (milk sugar) contained in milk. Some dogs, and more frequently, cats do not have the necessary digestive enzymes to handle this milk sugar. The result is fermentation and diarrhea. Your yogurt concoction undoubtedly contains considerable lactase, hence Dixie can handle it. For Dixie and other animals unable to digest milk sugar, the yogurt drink would prove superior nutritionally. For animals able to digest milk properly, the value received might depend more on price than profit."

What is "lactose" and why should any human being—or any dog or cat, for that matter—have trouble digesting it? Lactose is the not-very-sweet sugar in milk. Human milk contains 7 to 7½ percent lactose. Cow's milk is only 4½ percent lactose, which is the reason most baby formulas have some sweetening added to them to bring the sugar content up to that of human milk.

Since the main purpose of milk is to sustain the infant mammal, we must assume that lactose, the only carbohydrate in milk, provides energy, while the protein is used to build and repair cells. Scientists have reported that lactose also helps the body to absorb calcium. Unlike white sugar, which is absorbed immediately, lactose in absorbed very slowly in the intestines, and in the process establishes helpful intestinal bacteria which are capable of synthesizing a number of B vitamins. In parts of the world where there is little sunlight to provide vitamin D, the lactose prevents rickets and osteomalacia. Says *Dairy Council Digest* for September-October, 1974, "This suggests that lactose enhances calcium absorption as effectively as does vitamin D. It also helps the intestines to absorb protein."

When people who cannot digest lactose drink milk the lactose draws water from other parts of the body into the intestine and causes fermentation by colon bacteria, resulting in cramps, bloating, flatulence and diarrhea. This condition is called *lactose intolerance*. It occurs because there is none or too little of the enzyme *lactase* in that particular digestive tract.

There are three forms of this condition—congenital, primary and secondary. It seems some babies are born without the ability to digest lactose. This is an extremely rare and serious condition. It is believed to be caused by a mutation. Primary lactose intolerance is a condition in which newborns can drink milk with no trouble, but later in life they cannot. Secondary lactose intolerance involves a temporary condition due to degenerative or inflammatory disease, in which not just lactose but other sugars as well are not digested properly.

Less than 15 percent of all Scandinavians and Western European nationalities are unable to digest lactose. But about 60 to 80 percent of Greek Cypriots, American Indians, Arabs, Ashkenazi Jews, Mexican-Americans and American Blacks are unable to drink milk, and 90 percent of all Orientals and African Bantus are, we are told, unable to drink milk—that is, unable to digest milk sugar or lactose. Usually children lose their ability to drink milk between the ages of 2 and 12, depending on where they come from and what the milk-drinking patterns of their families were.

It seems reasonable to assume that all healthy mammals should be able to drink milk when they are born, since this is the food supplied by nature from their mothers' breasts. And it seems only natural that an enzyme, *lactase*, which helps the body to digest milk, should be present in newborn babies. It is. In cultures like the primitive Eskimos babies sometimes nurse for three or four years. The lactase processes the milk with no difficulty. But after an Eskimo baby is weaned, there is no chance that he will get any more milk, since Eskimos cannot raise herds of milk-producing animals. So, understandably, the lactase in his intestine would disappear since there is no further use for it.

This is, indeed, what happens in nations where dairy herds are not raised. The American Indians, early Chinese and Japanese people did not have cattle from which they could obtain milk, not because there is anything unhealthful about milk-drinking, but simply because their way of life or agriculture did not lend itself to dairying. So, presumably, their body supply of lactase disappeared soon after they were weaned.

When people from such a background come to the United States or Europe, where milk-drinking is widespread, they find they cannot digest milk. Because of this, some people have decided that milk is not good for all of us and they refuse to drink it. But an Oriental child, for example, raised in this country, who drinks cow's milk from the time he is weaned, will, other things being equal, be able to drink milk all his life, just as most Americans can. The lactase in his intestine remains there throughout life, since it is serving a metabolic purpose.

Reay Tannahill in *Food in History* tells us that if the early Chinese had not had such strong views on hygiene, they might have developed the soured milks which other nations have used for thousands of years—the yogurt, the Koumiss, the laban. But says Tannahill, "the Chinese may have classified soured milk as unclean or tainted. If so, they were wrong, for the chemistry of soured milk products makes them unusually hygienic."

The *lactobacillus* bacteria, which are in the "culture" with which yogurt and buttermilk are made, establish a very healthy condition in the colon, correct constipation and diarrhea, help the digestion of food and otherwise keep things in this department rolling along comfortably and well. And that is the reason why even cats and dogs, as well as human beings, can eat cheese and eat or drink yogurt, even if they lack the enzyme necessary to digest milk. If you or some member of your family has trouble digesting milk, try yogurt.

Whey is the liquid part of milk which separates out when

Nutrients in 100 Grams (About 3-1/2 Ounces) of Powdered Whey

Protein	13 grams
Lactose	73 grams
Calcium	646 milligrams
Phosphorus	589 milligrams
Thiamine	0.50 milligrams
Riboflavin	2.51 milligrams
Niacin	0.8 milligrams

Nutrients in One Cup of Yogurt Made of Partially Skimmed Milk

Protein	8 grams
Lactose	13 grams
Calcium	295 milligrams
Phosphorus	270 milligrams
Vitamin A	170 I.U.
Thiamine	0.1 milligrams
Riboflavin	0.4 milligrams
Niacin	0.2 milligrams

cheese is made. The solid part, the curds, go into the cheese. The liquid part, the whey, is produced in immense quantities by our cheese makers—29½ billion pounds in 1972. Until recently, nobody cared much about it and nobody did much to save the valuable nutrients it contains (see the accompaning chart). Dried or powdered whey is 13 percent protein, extremely rich in calcium and the B vitamins, especially riboflavin (B2), which is not very plentiful in other foods. It also contains about 74 percent lactose.

The U. S. Department of Agriculture experts believe that whey could go a long way toward meeting the demand for sweeteners, since, for every pound of protein in whey, there are eight pounds of lactose. They are also using it in a whey-soy beverage for overseas feeding programs. It is at least as nutritious as nonfat powdered milk.

Incidentally, if you should decide to take one of the lactobacillus products in pill form, which are available at your health food store, these take the place of yogurt, of course, by supplying the helpful bacteria in abundance. It is best always to take the tablets with some milk, to supply the lactose which is needed to encourage the growth of the helpful bacteria.

While on the subject of yogurt, however, we must report some disturbing news. Yogurt is one of the few foods left to us in the supermarket which you can feel absolutely safe in buying, if you stick to the unchemicalized, unsugared, unfruited, unflavored kinds.

Yogurt can and should consist of nothing but milk—either whole or skimmed with perhaps some powdered milk added—but in any case nothing but milk. PLUS—and this is the plus that makes the product—certain very healthful bacteria, mostly the *Lactobacillus acidophilus* or Lactobacillus Bulgaricus, which act very helpfully in the human intestine. These healthgiving bacteria—and there are billions of them in every tablespoon of yogurt—overcome all the pathogenic or harmful bacteria and help the human colon to achieve perfection.

Perfection, in this case, means smooth, trouble-free handling of waste material, so that we are scarcely aware of the function. It means correction of either constipation or diarrhea. It means rather rapid transit of wastes through the colon, so that they do not harden and become almost impossible to move. This rapid transit is also believed to help eradicate danger of colon cancer when we eat foods containing cancer-causing elements, as all of us must in the world in which we live.

The bacteria used to make yogurt give it the pleasant acid taste which most people find so appetizing. In recent years, mostly because of the enthusiasm of the health food movement, yogurt has become a most popular supermarket food. An article in *Food Technology* for November, 1975 tells us that sales of yogurt amounted to $125 million in 1974. The future for the yogurt industry looks bright, say the authors

---

Ever Wonder How Long Plain Yogurt Keeps Its Potency in Your Refrigerator?

"Yogurt has always been a fermented milk product containing billions of viable bacteria per gram. An investigation of commercial yogurt samples revealed the following ranges of total plate counts (of bacteria) per gram: 26 million to 4,159 million at the second day after purchase; 700 million to 30,300 million at the tenth day; and 1,200 million to 71,700 million at the 20th day. In all samples, the counts increased from day 2 to day 10 when held about 45 degrees F. in a walk-in refrigerator. In all samples except three, the counts continued to increase over the next ten days of storage."—*Food Technology*, November, 1975.

from Penn State University, Division of Food Science and Industry. So they did a survey to see just how many people eat yogurt and what they think of it in general.

The majority preferred fruit-flavored yogurt, they report, and most of them like the fruit all mixed up with the yogurt rather than at the bottom of the container. The surveyors asked the people they interviewed what they felt about "natural" yogurt. Over two-thirds said they prefer "natural" yogurt to one which contains synthetic additives, flavorings, dyes, preservatives and stabilizers.

And what about the bacteria it contains? Only 44 percent of all the people questioned know that yogurt contains bacteria. The rest eat yogurt, presumably, because they like it, because it's a "fun" thing and very fashionable, and because of its excellent nutritional value. A cup of yogurt contains all the nutrients of a cup of milk, plus the special bacteria. So, with their usual genius for going at things from the wrong end, food companies have sold the American public a "new" taste treat—yogurt. With goodness knows how much money spent on advertising, they have convinced a large segment of the population that they should eat yogurt.

Well and good. Nothing could make us happier. But now it seems—and why should it surprise us?—that the yogurt industry has decided to sell yogurt *without bacteria*. Believe it or not, that is the theme of this article in a trade magazine. By pasteurizing the yogurt at low heat, the manufacturers can retain the acid, tart taste but destroy all the bacteria so the product will keep for weeks or longer on supermarket shelves.

"As a matter of fact," says *Food Technology*, "both pasteurized and sterilized yogurt, with a much-prolonged shelf life—are already available. One major national brand is a pasteurized yogurt containing either no or relatively low numbers of bacteria. The question arises whether a consumer will be disappointed or feel cheated because the traditional expectation of massive numbers of bacteria was not satisfied by the pasteurized yogurt." Why shouldn't they feel cheated?

One reason is that 56 percent of yogurt-eaters studied apparently do not know that yogurt contains beneficial bacteria. They have been trained to believe that bacteria of any kind are "bad," so, presumably, any yogurt which boasts of having no bacteria should be the best to buy! But, aside from the protein, vitamins and minerals (the same as those of milk) and the sour taste, there is no reason to buy yogurt from which all the bacteria have been removed. You might as well buy plain milk for a lot less money.

The Powers That Be in Washington have a dilemma on their hands. They must, it seems, set up a "standard" for yogurt. For instance, they could rule that only yogurt containing the helpful bacteria can be labeled yogurt. Pasteurized yogurt would then have to be called artificial yogurt or something of the sort, which would supposedly warn the customer seeking helpful bacteria away from the product.

But most dairy products are consumed fairly near the place they are manufactured, because they are perishable. FDA regulations govern only products that cross state lines. So locally made yogurt would not have to use the FDA regulations. Unless state food laws demanded it, pasteurized yogurt would not have to be labeled as such. So the customer seeking the helpful bacteria of natural, unpasteurized yogurt, would not be able to tell whether the product on the shelf contained them or not.

The trick, of course, comes in the definition of yogurt. Says *Food Technology*, "One traditional view going back through the medical folklore of the last century and way back to Biblical times is that yogurt has therapeutic properties and that the presence of viable (living) bacteria is responsible for this benefit. The subject is still a controversial one since there is simply too much myth surrounding yogurt and too little scientific evidence to support the view."

It's true, of course, that making yogurt goes back to Biblical times and that, in many remote primitive countries today, a daily swig of a pint or more of yogurt is credited with achieving superlative health and longevity. It is also true that modern medical literature, especially in Eastern Europe, contains considerable reportage of carefully controlled laboratory experiments showing that yogurt bacteria are indeed helpful against many kinds of bacteria invasion. Certain Eastern European scientists are regularly treating cancer with yogurt, we understand.

The Food and Drug Administration, which will make the final decision, is chronically of the opinion that nothing in food has any relation to health, good or bad, except for certain well-delineated vitamin and mineral deficiencies which do not exist in the United States. So we can expect the FDA, acting in their traditional way, to declare that the bacteria in yogurt serve no purpose except to make the milk taste sour, so there is no need to indicate whether the stuff has been heated to destroy the bacteria. When that time comes, you, the health seeker, will have no choice but to make yogurt at home.

As for buying commercially made yogurt in a store, frankly, we don't know what to recommend. Read labels. If possible, don't buy pasteurized yogurt. It's cheaper to buy milk. If you can't find this kind of yogurt in a store and cannot make it at home, then give up yogurt for the time being—until the dilemma is resolved—or drink buttermilk (if you can find any that hasn't also been tampered with).

Destruction of jaw bones as we age accounts for loss of more teeth than we can credit to decay. Major gum problems, which the dentists call periodontal disease, herald this destruction. A well-known researcher in the field of calcium metabolism has found that merely by increasing calcium intake over long periods of time we can postpone or prevent this destruction of the bones which support our tooth and gum structure.

Dr. Leo Lutwak of Cornell University studied 80 adults with mild to severe periodontal disease. He gave part of the group 1,000 milligrams of calcium in the form of powdered milk, dicalcium phosphate or calcium gluconate, or calcium carbonate. He found steady increase in the density of the jaw bones in those who took the supplements for one year. There were no changes in the rest of the patients who had no supplements. Interestingly enough, there was no change in the blood or urine calcium in the people taking the supplements, meaning apparently that the mineral went right to work and was not excreted.

Before you begin to have troubles with loosening teeth and degenerating jaw bones, why not see that you get at least 1,000 milligrams of calcium every day? Dr. Lutwak believes that even more than this is advisable and will help to prevent osteoporosis in other parts of the body as well as the jawbones.

As mentioned a number of times in this book, osteoporosis is the disease in which bones become weak and brittle. A university specialist recently told a New York audience that osteoporosis is bound to become a growing problem, since the 50-plus age group is the fastest growing minority in the country.

Osteoporosis affects the entire skeleton. The back, the legs and feet are affected. As the spine collapses with time (because the small bones are too weakened to support it) the ribs may fall forward onto the rim of the pelvic bones, thus crowding all the digestive organs and creating much distress.

The disorder is largely responsible for the more than one million bone fractures each year in women over 40 years of age. "Seven hundred thousand of these occur in women with osteoporosis," said Dr. Louis V. Avioli, Professor of Medicine at Washington University in Missouri. "Seven hundred thousand of these fractures occur in women with osteoporosis, and 25 to 30 percent of all postmenopausal women have the ailment," he continued.

Osteoporosis is more common among women than men. The average man loses five to six percent of his bone mass every 10 years after the age of 35. At 65 bone loss slows to two to three percent every 10 years. In women the rate of loss is doubled. And 25 percent of American women of 40 are losing bone at a faster rate than other women their age.

A number of everyday things, including diet, are probably causes of bone loss, said Dr. Avioli, but not even the experts know which is the most important and why. Women have decreased levels of the sex hormone estrogen after menopause. This seems to be one reason for bone loss. (We would point out that recent research seems to show that taking estrogen in the form of a hormone pill may produce cancer, so it does not seem wise to try to replace the lost estrogen). Deficiency in calcium is undoubtedly another reason. And vitamin D is essential for the body to absorb calcium, as we discuss in more detail in the chapter on "Calcium."

Dr. Avioli mentions the importance of "muscle mass" which, he says, peaks at around 20 years of age. "The day-to-day pull on muscle tendons stimulates bone formation," he says. Inactivity also causes one to lose bone structure. The minerals just ease out of bones when we are confined to bed for long periods of time or when we spend most of the day sitting. This suggests that daily exercise is essential for maintaining healthy bones and avoiding osteoporosis.

And, as we have mentioned, it seems that there is a definite relationship between loss of bone and a diet in which there is too much protein in relation to calcium. If one is making use of dairy products which contain both protein and calcium, there seems to be no danger of this. But people who, for some reason, shun dairy products may eat lots of meat, which contains no calcium at all. Thus they throw the relationship out of balance. It is the acid-ash of the high meat diet which destroys the calcium level, according to Dr. Avioli. We would point out that a diet high in sugar also creates an acid-ash. So avoid the use of sugar if you would save your bone structure into a healthy old age.

Dr. Avioli tells us that about 6.3 million people in this country are at present suffering from acute problems relating to weakened bones in the spine. And eight million Americans have chronic problems related to the spine, compared to only

6 million in 1963. Our situation in regard to bone health is obviously getting worse year by year.

Then, too, recent surveys show, said the Missouri specialist, that a minimum of 10 percent of all women over 50 suffer from bone loss severe enough to cause hip, vertebrae or long-bone fractures.

"Surveys in homes for the aged and of ambulatory patients 50 to 95 years old have disclosed symptomatic back-pain osteoporosis in 15 and 50 percent of these populations respectively."

It's nothing to ignore, hoping that it won't happen to you as you grow older although you may have seen it happen to older relatives and friends. Dr. Avioli suggests the following means of prevention. Plenty of activity and exercise. Don't allow yourself to become house-bound or chair-bound or bedridden. Get out, move around, get interested in some hobby involving vigorous exercise.

Secondly, get enough calcium in diet and/or supplements. Can you get too much calcium? Apparently not, if other things are in good balance. Unwanted calcium deposits sometimes appear in various sites of the body. But this happens as often in those who are not getting enough calcium as in those who are getting enough, so it indicates some disturbance in the body mechanism which regulates calcium disposition in the body. The parathyroid gland, located near the thyroid gland in the throat, is in charge of this job. Some disorder in this gland can throw off the balance of blood calcium.

Mention of the thyroid gland brings us to the subject of another mineral, iodine. We generally think of iodine only as a mineral which, in extremely small amounts, is necessary for the health of this gland. The thyroid gland regulates many physiological activities of our bodies. It must have iodine to manufacture the thyroid hormone which it sends through the bloodstream to bring about many physical changes in our bodies.

Now there is evidence—and very important evidence it

seems to us—that lack of iodine in the diet may be a cause of cancer in women—cancer of the breast, the lining of the uterus and the ovaries. The theory is presented in *The Lancet* for April 24, 1976 by a scientist from the National Institute of Child Health and Human Development in Bethesda, Maryland.

Dr. Bruce V. Stadel bases his theory on figures of cancer incidence in various parts of the world. He reasons that this kind of cancer may be caused by something in the environment rather than being an inherited tendency. The incidence of breast cancer is higher among Japanese American women than among Japanese women living in Japan. And mortality rates for Japanese women living in our country are higher than those for Japanese women living in Japan, in regard to the three kinds of cancer listed above.

It is known that seaweed or kelp is eaten in Japan as a main part of the diet, along with a great deal of seafood. Both are rich sources of iodine. If Japanese women who come to the United States abandon these two foods and eat meals in which there is little iodine, this could account for the difference in cancer and mortality, if lack of iodine is indeed one of the causes of these diseases.

Another significant fact is that differences in breast-cancer rates in various parts of the United States and in various regions of the world parallel differences in the prevalence of goiter, which is a disease of iodine deficiency. Hence goiter and breast cancer are found much more frequently in the same geographical regions. Cancer of the lining of the uterus is also found more often in regions where goiter is found.

Says the author, "These observations suggest the hypothesis that environmental or genetic factors which increase the risk of goiter formation may increase the risk of breast, endometrial and ovarian cancer. Thus intake of the goitrogens (foods which cause goiter), or genetic abnormalities in iodine absorption and utilization and, most simply, a relatively low dietary iodine intake may be factors important in determining the risk of these cancers."

He goes on to describe how the thyroid gland controls the manufacture of various female hormones. In women with one or another of the cancers listed above, the balance of these hormones is off. The body is producing too much of some, too little of others. And because of the great influence of these hormones on tissues of the woman's breast, uterus and ovary, the effect of such an imbalance could well be cancer.

A relatively low dietary intake of iodine may produce borderline primary hypothyroidism, says Dr. Stadel. That is, a condition in which the thyroid gland is not working at its best, or is not doing all the job it was meant to do. "This state may not be obvious," he says, "either clinically or upon a single measurement of thyroid-hormone levels. At times during the reproductive life of affected women thyroid hormone levels may be normal, although likely to be at the lower end of normal." In other words, all the tests a doctor gives his woman patient may not be able to detect this slight deficiency in iodine which may later cause her such terrible difficulties with cancer. She may simply drag along with just a bit too little iodine and never know she lacks it. At some times in her life she may indeed get enough iodine, so that the thyroid gets back to normal operation for a while.

Dr. Stadel wants to test his theory. He outlines how he would go about it. Other researchers have already identified a large number of young women who are at high risk of breast cancer because it "runs in their families." These young women do indeed have the imbalances of female hormones which apparently accompany susceptibility to breast cancer.

Divide the group of young women into two groups, Dr. Stadel proposes. Advise one group to gradually increase their intake of iodine up to those levels found in Japanese women living in Japan. Continue to study the second group of women, but say nothing to them about increasing dietary iodine. Keep careful records on both groups of women, testing their female hormone level from time to time. If his hypothesis is correct, the scientist says the hormone imbalances should correct themselves in the women taking iodine, while the other group would notice no change. Part of the improvement in hormone balance would be correction of menstrual difficulties. Fertility should also increase.

"If this hypothesis is tested in the manner described above and the anticipated events occur, women in areas of the world where iodine intake is relatively low should be encouraged to increase their iodine intake," says Dr. Stadel.

We have no way of knowing whether or when such tests will be done. This need not influence our own course of action in regard to getting enough iodine every day to prevent imbalances in sex hormones as well as many other health catastrophes which can and do result from lack of iodine and disorders of the thyroid gland. A "goiter belt" is located in the central part of the United States—that part farthest from East and West seacoasts. Whatever iodine was in the soil originally has leached out of it over the centuries, so food grown there lacks iodine. In earlier days seafood was seldom available because it could not be imported over such long distances.

This was one of the reasons why salt is now iodized. If you are avoiding salt, then increase your diet of ocean fish. Then there is kelp, available in various forms at your health food store.

We mentioned the word "goitrogen" and we want to clarify this term, lest you become concerned that certain foods may be responsible for causing thyroid troubles. The *Cruciferae* family of plants contains a substance that is harmful to the thyroid gland if these foods are eaten in excessive amounts or if they are the only foods available to eat—as in the case of famines or war conditions.

This family of plants includes all the cabbage kin: cabbage, broccoli, Kohlrabi, Brussels sprouts, as well as garden cress and watercress, turnips, rutabaga, horseradish, mustard and several other plants not generally eaten in this country. This is one of the reasons we recommend eating a diet as widely varied as possible. Everything edible contains something that may prove harmful if you eat it in excess every day or if you eat it to the exclusion of all other foods.

Obviously nobody in his right mind would decide to live on horseradish or turnips. But we know of people, during the great wars in Europe, who lived for long periods of time on nothing but turnips, for there was nothing else to eat. They suffered from goiter as a result. But turnips and turnip greens are excellent food in a mixed diet and, in reasonable quantity, make a fine contribution to your meals. The same is true of all the other vegetables listed above.

Writing in the July 10, 1975 issue of the *Washington Post*, Dr. Jean Mayer says that people are using less and less iodized salt, so goiter from lack of iodine is beginning to appear in our country once again. Should we ask the government to order that all table salt be iodized? It seems not, for with all the other sources of iodine available, perhaps many people might get too much. And, on the other hand, lots of people, especially those with high blood pressure, are being put on low salt diets by their doctors. So they use little or no salt. If, at the same time they don't like seafood and are avoiding bread because of overweight or allergy, they might get almost no iodine at all!

If you do suffer from high blood pressure, your doctor has probably prescribed diuretics. These are drugs which increase urination. One of the reasons such drugs are prescribed is that they cause excess salt or sodium to be washed out of your bladder and excreted. Well and good. Most of us eat too much sodium—in the form of table salt—for our health.

But, eventually, if you continue to take the diuretic drugs you may begin to suffer from some bizarre symptoms: muscles may become weak and unreliable; you may have a "dragged out" feeling and the certainty that you simply cannot move one foot after the other. You may also have muscle cramps. These symptoms are indications that you are excreting too much potassium along with the sodium. And potassium, an essential mineral, must be carefully conserved by your body or you will suffer dire consequences eventually.

People not taking diuretics may also have trouble conserving enough potassium to assure healthy, well-functioning muscles. This group includes older folks, who tend always to be short on potassium; people with kidney disorders and people taking the heart drug digitalis. This is quite a large group to be threatened with deficiency in potassium.

Here are some suggestions from *Medical World News* for ways to get enough potassium and, at the same time, avoid foods high in sodium. If you are avoiding salt, you already know to eliminate all heavily salted foods like potato chips, pickles, olives, luncheon meats, many cheeses, bouillon cubes, catsup, caviar, commercial crackers, ham, herring, mustard, salted popcorn, salad dressings, salt pork, salted nuts, sausage, canned soups and other foods whose salty taste you can easily recognize.

But here are some foods which do not taste especially salty, but whose high salt content and low potassium content make them off-limits to the hypertensive on the low-salt diet, or taking diuretic drugs: canned tomato juice, raw clams, sardines, some commercial frozen foods that have been salted before they are frozen, such as lima beans and peas. Canned spinach and canned carrots are two other commercially available foods which contain considerable salt. So avoid them.

On the list of acceptable foods are those richest in potassium and containing the least sodium. These include the following:

Fruits: raw whole apples, apricots (canned, dried or fresh), avocado, bananas, cantaloupe, dried dates, grapefruit, nectarines, dried cooked prunes, raisins, watermelon.

Vegetables: asparagus in any form, all dried beans and lentils, fresh snap or green beans, Brussels sprouts, cabbage, cauliflower, corn on the cob, fresh lima beans, fresh peas, green peppers, baked or boiled potatoes, radishes, summer or winter squash. Bananas, raisins, potatoes and winter squash are especially rich in potassium.

Of fruit juices here are those which contain the most potassium: fresh or canned apple juice; grapefruit juice; prune juice; fresh, frozen or canned orange juice. Unsalted nuts or soybean snacks are also very rich in potassium. It goes without saying that you should not add any salt to any of these foods, either in the kitchen or at the table, if you are avoiding salt and trying to get as much potassium as possible.

If your doctor has placed you on a low-salt diet he has probably given you a salt substitute or recommended one. Some of these are herb mixtures which give foods a zesty taste without doing any damage to your salt balance. Others contain potassium in some form. Read the labels.

If you are shopping at the supermarket for fruit juices, don't make the mistake of buying one of the "fake" kinds which may boast about its vitamin C content, but which probably contains not one microgram of potassium, so you cannot depend on it to do for you what orange juice or grapefruit juice would do. What's wrong with buying oranges and grapefruit and squeezing the juice at home?

One final caution. Many people have water softeners in their homes or drink water softened at the community waterworks. The ion-exchange process used for removing the "hard" minerals—calcium and magnesium chiefly—substitutes sodium for these, so do not use softened water if you are on a low-salt diet. Softened water may be acceptable for a perfectly healthy person who does not eat too much salt. But for a person with high blood pressure, the salt in the drinking water could mean the difference between good health and soaring blood pressure figures.

If your home already has a water softener installed, ask your plumber to connect only the hot water to the flow of softened water. Then you can use only cold water for drinking and cooking. Or have your plumber install a spigot in some handy place before the water pipes enter the softener equipment. You can then draw water for drinking and cooking from this faucet.

New research is turning up exciting prospects for using the trace mineral chromium in conjunction with brewers yeast to stabilize the wild blood sugar swings of diabetics and, presumably, victims of low blood sugar as well. Dr. Richard J. Doisy, a biochemist at the State University of New York Upstate Medical School Center in Syracuse, believes it is likely that "public health measures to ensure adequate chromium intake will be not only desirable but essential for the longrange health of this nation."

Is seems that the trace mineral chromium, which is essential to human beings in very small or "trace" amounts, may soon be used to prevent and to treat the diabetes so common among older Americans and possibly also the raised levels of fats in their blood. It is believed that lack of enough insulin may be responsible for the accumulation of these fats. And, if chromium can be used to potentiate—that is, to make more powerful—the available insulin, then perhaps the fatty accumulations can be prevented.

Dr. Doisy has been testing elderly Americans for their chromium content. He found that they have far less chromium in their bodies than people of a like age in the Middle East, the Far East and in more primitive nations in Africa. And, along with the lack of chromium goes the impairment of blood sugar regulating machinery which is controlled by insulin. Insulin, you will remember, is the hormone secreted by the human gland, the pancreas. If the pancreas cannot produce enough insulin to process the starches and sugars eaten by an individual, that person will probably succumb to diabetes.

Dr. Doisy and his colleagues have found that lack of chromium is not confined to the elderly people. Even among much younger patients, Dr. Doisy found that giving chromium improved what is called "glucose tolerance" as well as lowering the blood levels of cholesterol and other fats. Glucose tolerance is the ability of the body to process correctly sugars and starches.

A researcher at the University of Colorado Medical Center used hair samples to chart the blood levels of chromium in people of various ages. He found, according to *Medical World News* for October 11, 1974, that, after the first few months of life, babies showed a drop in the level of chromium in their blood. Women having babies had much less chromium in their blood after the child was born. He found that Americans of all ages are not getting enough chromium.

Dr. Doisy studied elderly people living in a housing project in Syracuse. Of 31 active healthy people over 63, almost half had disorders of glucose tolerance—that is, impairment of their body's ability to deal successfully with sugar and starchy foods. Twelve of these people agreed to take brewers yeast. Within a month, half of them had normal glucose tolerance. Their cholesterol levels also dropped from an average of 245 milligrams to 205 milligrams.

Debittered Brewers Yeast Approximate Analysis

Protein	50%
Carbohydrate	31%
Fat	5.8%
Calories per gram	3.5
Calcium	1.25%
Phosphorus	1.5%
Potassium	1.62%
Magnesium	0.25%
Sodium	0.22%
Copper	8.5 ppm
Iron	55 ppm
Zinc	45 ppm
Manganese	6.5 ppm

* ppm—parts per million

Of course, brewers yeast contains another substance which is known to reduce cholesterol levels—the B vitamin niacin. But for this you need large amounts of niacin (B3). Dr. Doisy believes his volunteers were not getting enough of this vitamin from the yeast supplement to be responsible for the abrupt drop in cholesterol. It must be the chromium along with a factor which is found in brewers yeast called Glucose Tolerance Factor (GTF), which seems to make the chromium more available to the body.

Children apparently can use chromium much more successfully than older folks. The older folks did not respond to chromium for several months. But when they took the GTF factor in yeast along with the chromium they responded within a month. So it seems that the ability of the body to convert chromium into a usable substance declines with age. Some of Dr. Doisy's diabetic patients have reported that the GTF in brewers yeast has stabilized their blood sugar levels and has prevented attacks of low blood sugar which, in a diabetic, can be very serious.

Another interesting fact turned up in Dr. Doisy's research. We know this will interest health seekers who campaign against white sugar and all foods that contain it. Dr. Doisy found that giving his patients large amounts of sugar brought about excessive excretion of chromium. Such a finding reveals the fact that white refined sugar can damage the susceptible person in two ways, as regards blood sugar levels. First, practically all the chromium that is present in sugar cane is removed when the sugar is refined. So the person who eats white sugar must somehow deal with it, without the help of the trace mineral chromium, which accompanies it in the natural form of sugar cane. Now we discover that eating white sugar alone causes the body to excrete whatever chromium it has, which makes the situation far, far worse. No wonder so many Americans are deficient in chromium when so large a part of their diet is white sugar and foods that contain it.

The Glucose Tolerance Factor which enables the body to

B Vitamins in One Gram of Brewers Yeast

(One gram is less than half a teaspoon)

micrograms

Vitamin B1 (Thiamine)	150
Vitamin B2 (Riboflavin)	50
Vitamin B3 (Niacin)	400
Vitamin B6 (Pyridoxine)	40
Pantothenic acid	100
Biotin	1.25
Choline	3350
Inositol	4425
Folic Acid	5

use chromium easily and effectively is present in brewers yeast in more abundance than in any other food. It is also present in liver, kidney, mushrooms and several spices. Of course, we eat spices in extremely small amounts so they could not be used as a good source for this factor. Foods which contain lots of chromium, relatively speaking—for chromium exists in extremely small amounts in food—are these: wheat germ and bran, wholewheat, wholegrains of all kinds, nuts, natural fats rather than highly processed ones and, of course, brewers yeast. For additional information about GTF, refer to our earlier chapter on "Chromium."

An editorial in *The Lancet*, March 6, 1976 points out once again the importance of magnesium to good health and the various kinds of dietary imbalances or conditions of ill health that can lead to deficiency. Those of us who get large amounts of calcium without regard to our magnesium intake may be courting deficiency, for a high calcium intake seems to necessitate a rather high magnesium intake. Dairy products, which are an excellent source of calcium, are poor sources of magnesium. Seed foods and cereals, which are the best sources of magnesium, are poor sources of calcium. So the best idea is a good balance of the two.

Symptoms of gross magnesium deficiency may be convulsions, depression, vertigo, ataxia (difficulty in walking) and muscle weakness. Giving magnesium quickly brings things back to normal if deficiency is the cause.

One common cause of magnesium deficiency is prolonged loss of fluids from the digestive and intestinal tract without replacing them. This might occur in vomiting or diarrhea disorders. There may also be magnesium loss in renal failure and in the presence of glandular disorders such as over- or under-activity of the parathyroid gland. Alcoholics and patients on long-term intravenous therapy are likely to suffer from lack of magnesium. Heart and high blood pressure patients taking diuretics are usually aware of the dangers of potassium loss, as we have reported. But losses of magnesium are also likely and should be carefully watched for by anyone taking diuretics for any length of time.

In some heart conditions, diuretic therapy along with other complicating conditions may produce quite serious magnesium deficiency, which can cause irregular heart beats and precipitate digitalis toxicity in the same way that potassium deficiency does.

Many doctors believe that lack of magnesium in the water supply may explain the higher incidence of circulatory disorders in localities where the water is "soft," hence lacking in this mineral.

Relief of magnesium deficiency is only hours away if one takes a magnesium supplement. Since there is little danger of getting too much, it seems wise to add magnesium to one's daily supplements if any of the above conditions seem imminent.

Kidney stones and bladder stones made up chiefly of calcium oxalate or a mixture of calcium phosphate "present a stubborn and curious puzzle to the urologist," says a review in the January, 1976 issue of *Nutrition Reviews*. There just doesn't seem to be much reason why certain individuals should suffer from these painful disorders, since they appear to be otherwise healthy and the amount of calcium in their blood appears to be "normal."

Symptoms of both kinds of stones are: pain and frequent, bloody urination. Small stones may pass out through the ureter. Larger stones which may block the flow of urine must be removed by surgery or some other method. Up to now, specialists have generally believed that bladder stones are caused by chronic inflammation of the bladder, enlargement of the male prostate gland, contraction of the neck of the bladder, a diverticulum or pouch in the wall of the bladder or kidney stones which have moved down into the bladder.

Now we are told in *Nutrition Reviews* that stones may be caused by deficiency in an important mineral and an equally important vitamin. The mineral is magnesium. The vitamin is vitamin B6 or pyridoxine. A lengthy experiment involving some 150 people seems to show great improvement in the tendency to form such stones when people who are susceptible are given the two nutrients over a long period of time.

The experiment was accomplished by getting the aid of a large number of urologists who agreed to give the two nutrients to a given number of patients who could be expected to form a given number of stones in the time of the experiment—five years. About 150 patients were involved. Certain qualifications were set. Only patients who had formed at least one stone in the previous five years were accepted. They must also be free from urinary infection, have normal kidney function, normal levels of calcium and phosphorus in the blood and be free from other diseases which sometimes accompany stone formation—peptic ulcer, for example.

The volunteers were given a magnesium supplement consisting of 100 milligrams three times a day. By this we assume they took the tablets with meals. They were also given 10 milligrams of vitamin B6 daily. No other change was made in diet or treatment.

The reduction in stone formation was dramatic. The group

as a whole had formed an average of 1.3 stones before they began treatment. Taking the food supplements for five years resulted in an average of only one-tenth of a stone during the five years the test continued. Furthermore, the only stones formed were limited to 17 of the 150 subjects. The others had no stones at all during this five-year period. None of them suffered any side effects.

The *Nutrition Reviews* writer professes amazement at these results. What could they mean? he asks. Is it possible that the person who regularly forms kidney or bladder stones has a marginal deficiency in magnesium and/or pyridoxine, either because he doesn't get enough at mealtime or because he just happens to need more than the average person? We would say, gentlemen, that both of these circumstances may certainly be the reason for formation of stones. Magnesium and pyridoxine are both found most abundantly in wholegrain cereals and breads as well as other seed foods. When white flour is made, most of the magnesium and vitamin B6 are discarded and never replaced in the flour. Why should not modern human beings be short on both nutrients?

But, says the *Reviews* writer, these people did not seem to be suffering from a magnesium deficiency. And, what is more, people who are known to be suffering from a magnesium deficiency, as a result of lack of absorption, prolonged diarrhea, excessive alcohol intake or protein malnutrition, do not generally form stones.

In the case of pyridoxine, there seems to be even less evidence of a deficiency. In fact, it seems that the pyridoxine may not be necesssary to the success of such a trial. An earlier experiment showed that magnesium supplements alone stopped the formation of stones in the people tested.

The article goes on to tell us that in laboratory rats on a diet low in magnesium bladder stones are *always* found. Calcium oxalate stones are *always* found in laboratory rats on a diet low in vitamin B6. A strongly alkaline urine and a reduced excretion of magnesium will produce stones.

A diet low in magnesium, but high in phosphorus and moderate in calcium tends to cause stone formation in kidneys and heart. This kind of diet is probably widespread in our country, for meat is high in phosphorus, which tends to overbalance the lack of magnesium (found mostly in cereal foods and bread). When all the breads and cereals you eat have had their magnesium removed, the balance between the two minerals would be thrown out of kilter.

The question of why some otherwise healthy people tend to form stones while others do not, and why the addition of magnesium and pyridoxine should stop the stone formation remains a mystery, says *Nutrition Reviews*. But there is valuable evidence that this is so. Since the therapy is completely harmless this study "should encourage its wider application," says the magazine.

Nutrition Reviews is published by the Nutrition Foundation, a trade organization of the giant food industry. It is the official position of this industry that the American food supply is totally adequate in all respects and that it is totally impossible for any American eating "the average American diet" to be deficient in any nutrient. So one would expect that their publication would be unable to explain how two simple, essential nutrients, given in rather large amounts, might correct a long-standing disorder as serious as stone formation.

However, we "food faddists" have known for years that many of us may be deficient in many nutrients, both because we cannot get enough of them at our daily meals and because we, as individuals, may have needs for individual nutrients far higher than "the average."

In his book, *Vitamin B6, the Doctor's Report*, Dr. John Ellis shows the relationship between magnesium and pyridoxine. He relates stories of his patients who suffered from a variety of disorders which yielded to magnesium and vitamin B6 supplements.

One is perfectly safe in taking far more pyridoxine than the 10 milligrams these doctors gave their patients. Many specialists are now requesting that this B vitamin be included regularly in all contraceptive pills, since it appears that women taking these pills are bound to be short on pyridoxine. Many other conditions of ill health are seemingly related to shortage of vitamin B6, due largely, one must believe, to its almost total absence from those foods which make up half the meals of many people—white sugar and white flour and everything made from them.

Dr. David L. Earnest of the University of California in San Francisco believes that people who are unable to absorb fat properly may be susceptible to kidney stones because the fat in such a person's intestine tends to unite with most of the calcium there, hence robbing the body of its essential calcium.

One of the functions of calcium is to unite with oxalates in food, rendering them harmless. The more calcium available, the less danger there is that oxalates (or oxalic acid) will cause any trouble. This is the reason we recommend lots of calcium at meals, especially if one eats a lot of spinach, rhubarb and other foods that contain considerable oxalic acid. Plenty of calcium protects against any possible harm from the oxalates.

But people who suffer from Crohn's Disease, non-tropical sprue, pancreatic insufficiency and other conditions where fat is not absorbed may lose most of their calcium to the unabsorbed fat in their digestive tracts. This frees the oxalate and allows it to be absorbed through the intestinal wall rather than being excreted in the feces. It is then carried to the kidney and excreted in urine. If there is a large amount of it in the urine, it may unite there with whatever calcium is present and form kidney stones.

The remedy, says Dr. Earnest, is to give large doses of calcium or aluminum or lanthanum, which is a rare earth metal that precipitates oxalates. At the San Francisco General Hospital, Dr. Earnest gave four grams of calcium (that's 4,000 milligrams) a day to patients who habitually showed oxalic acid in their urine. This reduced the oxalic acid and did not increase the calcium in the urine. Extra calcium was excreted in the stool.

In those patients who had high levels of calcium in their urine, he gave aluminum hydroxide which also reduced the oxalic acid in their urine, but caused other trouble in the form of lost phosphorus. By giving a nightly dose of phosphorus, Dr. Earnest corrected this situation and kept the expected kidney stones from forming.

It is difficult, he says, to discover just how much oxalic acid is present in American foods. We know that spinach and other leafy greens contain considerable amounts of oxalic acid. But they also contain considerable calcium, so they should not cause any trouble, if eaten in moderation, since, in healthy people, the calcium will combine with the oxalates and render them harmless.

But, says Dr. Earnest, "aside from spinach and rhubarb, there's an incredibly small amount of information on the oxalate content of American foods. Who knows what's in a hot dog?" One of his patients who was on a diet from which all oxalic acid containing foods had been carefully removed was still excreting oxalates in his urine. Testing the cola beverage this patient was drinking, the researchers found a sizable quantity (8 milligrams) in the soft drink.

Another specialist in this field, Dr. Frederic L. Coe of Chicago, expressed his delight at these simplified methods of treating the tendency to form kidney stones. "Very exciting results," he called them. And he said that the idea of using the earth metal lanthanum for precipitating oxalate is "fantastically interesting and extremely important." This story appeared in *Medical World News* for September 6, 1976.

News of still another development in kidney stone research turned up in the *British Medical Journal* for July 10, 1976. It seems that certain ethnic groups in some nations are virtually the only people in those nations who suffer from kidney stones. In Fiji, the Indians, who came originally from the Indian subcontinent, make up about half the population and are the only people who ever get kidney stones. They come from widely varied family backgrounds, so apparently this tendency to form stones is not inherited.

"The explanation may be a matter of diet," says the *BMJ* editorial. These folks were found to have no abnormalities in the way their bodies handle calcium, uric acid and amino acids. And there is nothing to suggest any inborn dysfunction of the kidneys. They may get stones for the same reason other East Indians have been found to be susceptible—large amounts of peppery, hot, spicy foods at meals. A physician has found that five of his patients had evidence of severe kidney damage, some of them had stones.

The traditional diet of these people is rich in curries and spices. That is, these folks eat curry, spices or pickles in some form every day. One physician estimated that Fijian Indians must eat about the equivalent of one bottle of Worcestershire sauce every day in curries. In addition, ginger and cinnamon are used in large amounts.

The *BMJ* writer calls their disease "curry kidney." He asks if someone might examine the health and diet of East Indians in other countries—England, for example—to see if their consumption of hot spices and their susceptibility to kidney disorders may match that of the Fiji Indians.

The lesson seems clear. Hot, peppery foods should be eaten in very small quantities, if at all. They should not make up a major part of one's diet. Their volatile oils may threaten the kidneys which, after all, have to excrete all that remains of these peppery substances. A dash of this or that adds agreeable piquancy to many foods, especially if one must eat little or no salt.

But in some parts of the world peppery hot herbs are used in large quantities. No one has ever been able to point to any benefit these spices bring except to hide the taste of spoiled food. This was the reason spices had such great value in ancient times. With no refrigeration, most foods that contained any fat were rancid by the time they got to the table. So ancient cooks, from Greek and Roman times on through all European history, laid on the spices with a heavy hand. And in hot countries today where refrigeration is not available, spices are used to conceal the taste of spoiled food. In our country, we have no need for such seasonings. Fresh food is easily available. Home refrigeration is almost universal. Let's be careful to be guided, in all things, by moderation. Too much of anything is not good.

A physician from Seattle has been treating arthritic patients with a daily zinc supplement given with each of the day's three meals. He reports that results have been encouraging.

The Lancet for September 11, 1976 contains an article by Dr. Peter A. Sinkin of Seattle describing a trial of zinc supplements for 24 of his patients with "refractory" rheumatoid arthritis. This means arthritis which did not respond to any other method of treatment. It was a double-blind experiment.

That is, the volunteers were divided into two groups. One group was given their regular medication plus zinc supplements for 12 weeks. The others got their regular medication plus a tablet which contained nothing. Not until the end of the trial, when all observations on joint swelling, morning stiffness, walking time had been made and the patients themselves described how they felt, was the code broken so that patients and doctors alike knew which had received the zinc supplement.

The doctor examined all patients at the beginning of the trial, recording scores for swelling of joints, tenderness in each joint, along with scores for the length of time morning stiffness persisted, and grip strength, as well as ability to walk 50 feet in less than 30 seconds. Patients reported any symptoms they had of such things as discomfort, nausea, vomiting, change in appetite or bowel habits and so forth. X-rays of all hands were taken at the beginning of the test, again in 24 weeks.

Says Dr. Sinkin, "patients taking zinc sulfate fared better in all clinical parameters than did patients receiving placebo (the nothing pill)." In every area investigated—swelling, pain, stiffness, walking time, the ones getting the mineral improved while those who did not take the zinc showed little or no improvement. The only test in which the zinc did not seem to bring much improvement was the grip strength. An early improvement in the test group was not sustained, says Dr. Sinkin.

After the original test, all the volunteers in both groups were given zinc supplements and all reported improvement. There were few side effects. Headache, rash, change in appetite, abdominal pain or discomfort and diarrhea were all reported oftener in the group not getting the zinc supplement than in the group which got it. All side effects were mild, however.

The zinc sulfate was taken after meals to prevent any difficulties with nausea. Dr. Sinkin suggests that it would be preferable to take a zinc supplement which would be better absorbed and would be taken without any digestive irritation. "From our experience," he says, "and that of others, virtually all patients can tolerate oral zinc sulfate for three to six months. Possible toxic effects of prolonged use must still be carefully sought." He believes that much additional work must be done to confirm his observations and to determine what part zinc plays in the health of joints.

If you suffer from arthritis, there is no reason to delay in taking a zinc supplement. There is no need to take the sulfate form which Dr. Sinkin gave to his patients. Your health food store has zinc supplements which are readily absorbed. These come in various potencies, marked on the label. An especially valuable kind is the "chelated" product, meaning that the mineral has been associated with amino acids which "chelate" it into a form which is much more readily absorbed by the body.

Dr. Sinkin's patients were taking large amounts of zinc three times daily. Much more zinc would undoubtedly be absorbed from a chelated product than from the zinc sulfate tablet which Dr. Sinkin gave. So there seems to be no need to take as much as he was giving patients in his experiment. Eat lots of those foods which contain plenty of zinc and avoid those from which it has been removed. And take a zinc supplement. It is a perfectly natural substance which cannot harm you.

It's hard to imagine a more difficult or discouraging disease to treat than one called *acrodermatitis enteropathica*. Fortunately it is rare. Unfortunately, it is apparently sometimes inherited. It brings terrible blistering sores on the skin, sores on the mucus membranes of mouth and throat, diarrhea and loss of hair. Usually it occurs in infants when they are taken off breast milk and given formulas.

Drugs which have been used are sometimes successful. If they are not, the baby must be kept on breast milk, no matter how this is arranged. If untreated, says an article in the *New England Journal of Medicine* for April 24, 1975, the disease is usually fatal, though some victims have survived and have apparently outgrown this inherited defect, although we have been told that inherited defects usually persist throughout life.

Quite recently the trace mineral zinc has been used to treat this disorder and patients have responded "dramatically." The *Journal* article describes still another patient, this one a 22-year-old woman who developed the disease when she was only three months old. When she was 1½ years old she was at the point of death when her life was saved by drugs which she had to take every day. For some reason the drug increased the amount of zinc in her blood. Several years ago this observation led to doctors giving zinc to see what the effects would be.

In this case, as in earlier ones, the effects were startling and gratifying. This woman had had two pregnancies which ended in spontaneous abortions. Then she had a stillborn defective child. Since then she has taken The Pill.

The doctors at a Colorado hospital gave her first the drug which usually controlled her condition. Then they withheld it until ominous symptoms began to appear. Blisters began to form on her knees, her mouth tissues became sore and she began to feel ill and depressed.

They gave her zinc sulfate—220 milligrams three times a day—and she responded rapidly and dramatically. Within 24 hours she felt well. Within four days her skin blisters and other symptoms had completely disappeared. Levels of zinc in her blood became normal. The doctors stopped the treatment after ten days and she remained well without any treatment. But within five weeks symptoms had returned and the zinc levels in her blood were once again low.

On zinc therapy—100 milligrams this time, given in two daily doses, she improved once again—showing improvement within 24 hours. The doctors believe, they say, that her response to this trace mineral indicates that this disease is very much involved with the metabolism of zinc. Either the patient cannot absorb enough zinc to keep her healthy or she loses it before it can do her any good. The amount finally needed to keep her well is, they comment, only a little above the recommended daily allowance for zinc, which is 15 milligrams. The 100 milligrams of zinc sulfate contain about 22 milligrams of zinc.

Severe zinc deficiency could explain all the symptoms of this unpleasant and serious disorder. Animals made deficient in zinc have retarded growth. They lack appetite, they suffer from skin disorders and loss of hair; the area around their fingernails becomes infected, their sexual organs do not develop properly. They become lethargic and are very susceptible to infections. Offspring of animal mothers which are deficient in zinc have abortions and congenitally malformed offspring. In many human beings the sense of taste is lost during zinc deficiency. There also seems to be some defect in handling some of the food fats in people who are deficient in zinc.

We were impressed recently with some material on zinc by Robert Rodale, the son of J. I. Rodale. He has done lots of research on the subject and covers it in very understandable form in his book, *The Best Health Ideas I Know*, which was published by Rodale Press, Emmaus, Pa.

Rodale says there is lots of evidence that we need far more zinc than the present estimate for a daily allowance. One of the main reasons may be that the zinc content of our food is declining all the time because of the use of modern commercial fertilizers which provide no zinc. Yields on grain are increasing because of all the fertilizer our farmers use, but the zinc content of soils is dropping, not only in this country but also in many parts of the world.

He tells us that a group of Colorado children were found to be quite short on zinc, as indicated by slow growth rates and severe deficiencies in the senses of taste and smell. Another specialist in the field points out that vegetarians may suffer most from zinc deficiency. This mineral is needed for the body to use protein. It is most abundant in high protein foods like meat and fish. So vegetarians who use no animal products may lack zinc, even though they get enough protein in their vegetarian foods. They cannot use all this protein without enough zinc to process it. And vegetarian foods may be especially lacking in zinc due to lack in the soils in which the food is grown.

Two Midwestern scientists, Dr. Donald F. Caldwell and Dr. Donald Oberleas, believe that as many as 80 percent of all Americans may be deficient in zinc. Our bodies lose zinc in excretions when we have colds, also in perspiration. Zinc is lost, too, when foods are processed. Even canning and cooking cause some loss of zinc. But most important is the amount lost when cereal foods and sugar are refined, and made into white flour, processed cereals and white sugar.

Dr. William Strain and Dr. Walter Pories are two scientists working constantly on zinc studies. They have found that the trace mineral helps to heal wounds, decreases pains in the legs of people suffering from intermittent claudication, a circulatory ailment, and possibly helps to prevent hardening of the arteries.

Here are some symptoms which may be linked to deficiency in zinc, although other conditions may be involved as well: lethargy, apathy and unwillingness to learn, according to a psychologist. Lack of ability to use all protein in the diet, since zinc is involved in this process. According to Dr. Jean Mayer, formerly of Harvard, zinc also helps one to recover from fatigue caused by exercise and helps undo the effects of alcohol.

Drs. Strain and Pories found that people suffering from hardening of the arteries were deficient in zinc. Giving zinc supplements brought some dramatic benefits to such patients. Two Tennessee doctors reported rapid healing of gums after tooth extraction when zinc was given. More than 30 different enzyme systems in the body depend on zinc as one of their ingredients—about three times more than are dependent on magnesium. Enzyme systems are those groups of nutrients—proteins, hormones, vitamins and minerals—which bring about chemical changes in our bodies, allowing us to utilize food and build it into our cells or use it as energy.

"No part of the human anatomy contains more zinc than the prostate gland," says Robert Rodale. "Actually a healthy man has several times more zinc in his prostate than he does in most other soft tissues of his body." He goes on to tell us that large doses of zinc have improved prostate health in experiments conducted in Chicago. Scientists found that seven percent of all men they tested have low levels of zinc in their semen and 30 percent are borderline. They have given zinc to men suffering from chronic prostatitis (not caused by bacterial infection), have gotten good results in 70 percent of these.

If zinc is obviously essential and involved in so much that goes on inside us, why are not doctors more concerned about it and why do they not give their patients zinc supplements? Rodale lists some reasons. Doctors are notoriously uninterested in nutrition. The typical American diet, which is causing zinc deficiency, is thought by most doctors to be the best possible diet. Then, too, giving trace minerals is a way to prevent disease, rather than healing a condition already present. Doctors are looking for quick cures for acute diseases, mostly. They seldom express much interest in preventing disease, except by vaccination.

Zinc therapy is not an overnight therapy. As is the case with any nutritional therapy, it works slowly. It may take quite a long time to undo the damage done over many years by inadequate diet. Zinc is a common mineral, which cannot be patented or sold as an expensive drug. So drug companies are not much interested in promoting it. They can't make much money out of it. Doctors get much, if not most, of their information on therapy from drug salesmen and drug advertising.

And most doctors—like most official spokesmen on nutrition—believe that no patient is short on zinc unless he comes in half-dead from well-recognized symptoms of zinc deficiency. Not many of us in this country ever show such definite symptoms. But this does not mean we are getting optimum amounts of zinc for good health.

One specialist in zinc metabolism believes adults should be getting up to 25 milligrams daily. Dr. Harold Rosenberg in his book, *The Doctor's Book on Vitamin Therapy*, published by G. P. Putnam's Sons, New York, recommends up to 30 milligrams. Supplements of higher potency are available only on prescription. These are generally zinc sulfate, zinc gluconate, zinc chloride. Zinc carbonate, which seems most acceptable, since it is a natural product which is mined, is not yet available as a supplement for human beings, although it is used in animal feed. Bone meal contains zinc in natural form, but not a great deal in terms of the potencies we are talking about here.

So your first concern should be to get as much zinc from meals as you possibly can. Fish and shellfish contain more zinc than any other foods. Oysters are abundant sources. Liver, beef, egg yolk, brewers yeast are other excellent sources. Wholewheat cereal and bread have not had their zinc removed by processing, so they contribute considerable amounts to your diet. White bread and processed supermarket cereals are all but useless as sources.

"Crib death" or Sudden Infant Death Syndrome (SIDS)

kills perhaps 20,000 American babies every year. This cruel drama takes its toll of young parents as well, many of whom are unjustly suspected of being responsible for the baby's death, many of whom assume unwarranted guilt and blame themselves, thinking they must have done something wrong.

The perfectly healthy baby is put to bed, cooing and smiling. His mother comes to check on him during the night, or the next morning and finds him dead, with no sign of a struggle or any convulsive movements. Physicians and researchers have suggested many causes. Most of them seem to be related to the completely unnatural conditions that surround most American babies from the very moment of birth.

Dr. Mavis Gunther, a British physician, theorizes in the February 22, 1975 issue of *The Lancet* that "cot deaths" as they are called in England, result from infections or allergies induced in the baby by bottle-feeding. Her reasoning is that all mammalian young refuse any kind of food except their mother's milk during an appropriate period after birth. It is well known to scientists that breast milk contains resistance factors which protect the baby from infections until he is old enough to develop his own protective mechanism.

"The effectiveness of breast feeding in defense against viral and bacterial infection has only tardily been accepted, but it is real," says Dr. Gunther. The first milk after childbirth, called colostrum, is known to be very rich in protective factors but so, too, is breast milk later on. Certainly bottle-fed babies are more liable to infection. Some pediatricians believe this is because the mechanics of bottle-feeding lend themselves to contamination with bacteria. But in animals as well as human beings vital protection against an array of disorders is guaranteed by mother's milk, whereas cow's milk contains no such protection for human babies.

Rabbits that are raised in germ-free environments and fed on cow's milk die when they are 18-22 days old, says Dr. Gunther, at an age when behavior ordinarily makes mammary feeding obligatory and nibbling on other food is only starting. In the case of the rabbits, as in human babies, death may be caused by bacteria to which the infant has not developed immunity or to some allergen to which he is susceptible.

Most babies which die of crib death are bottle-fed. The risk is much greater also in babies whose weight at birth was too low. The incidence is much higher, too, among young mothers who have had children in quick succession without access to highly nutritious diets. So lack of protein and lack of folic acid, a B vitamin, are suspected as one more reason for such tragedies. Babies dying this way generally have watery accumulations in their lungs, suggesting that they could not get enough oxygen to keep breathing normally.

In the same issue of *The Lancet* comes word from another British source that lack of vitamin E and the trace mineral selenium may have something to do with crib deaths. Vitamin E does not pass freely from mother to unborn baby, say Drs. E. Tapp and C. Anfield of Manchester. Human babies are born with much lower levels of vitamin E in their blood than adults have. They may develop a kind of anemia as a result. The levels of vitamin E in the blood rise much more slowly in infants given formulas than in those who are breast-fed. A study of 14 infants dying of crib death showed in general much lower levels of vitamin E than in those babies who died of other conditions.

And from New Zealand, in November, 1971 evidence reached us from an Animal Health Laboratory that human babies are being raised under conditions of deficiency in both selenium and vitamin E, which would not for a moment be tolerated in animal husbandry. Says Dr. F. C. Money, autopsies of the victims of crib death show the same conditions found in animals dead from lack of vitamin E and selenium. "Many fatal vitamin E and/or selenium deficiency diseases of the young of about 40 mammalian and bird species are known," he says. Most deaths occur only when both nutrients are lacking, since one can substitute for the other.

Found at autopsies are hemorrhages from small blood

vessels in the lungs and adjacent chest walls, filling of the lungs with blood fluid, degenerative changes of, and hemorrhages in the vital heart muscle and hemorrhages around the spinal cord. When there is not enough oxygen, Dr. Money says, "the normal oxidative processes by which tissues gain their energy and heat, extend into the tissues themselves where chain reaction proceeds unchecked. Simply this means that otherwise healthy tissues combust. The reaction is termed peroxidation and in prevention of this, vitamin E acts as an antioxidant."

Dr. Money goes on to describe other conditions of infants, such as *retrolental fibroplasia*, which causes blindness. It can be prevented by vitamin E. This disorder occurred in many premature infants exposed to too high a concentration of oxygen in their incubators, long before anyone suspected what was causing these tragedies.

Consumer Bulletin for June, 1972 tells us that cow's milk is deficient in vitamin E and high in phosphates which the baby's kidneys have trouble dealing with. In human milk there is considerably more vitamin E and it is in proper balance with the unsaturated fats. This is important, since getting too much of these fats tends to raise one's needs for vitamin E. The *Bulletin* tells us that guinea pigs fed a diet deficient in vitamin E showed many of the same conditions, after death, that infants dying of crib death show.

A disease of newborn infants called Respiratory Distress Syndrome may be caused by lack of lecithin in their lungs, according to a group of Welsh physicians who reported their findings in *Nature* for February 25, 1972. This is a disease which kills babies within a few days after birth. Tests on 97 infants showed that those who were delivered in good health had lecithin levels of 3.5 to 37.5. Of 13 infants who developed the respiratory disease lecithin levels were only 0.6 to 3.4. In every case the lowest level of lecithin accompanied the most severe respiratory distress.

Breast milk is a mixture of many things, including lecithin and cholesterol, as well as trace minerals, B vitamins, vitamin

A, vitamin C, and the minerals calcium and phosphorus. Now we learn that it contains much larger amounts of vitamin E than does cow's milk. Everyone who makes official statements in the field of pediatrics admits that no one can reproduce breast milk, no matter how hard they try. It's simply too complex a mixture, so there is no way of knowing how many other essential elements we are leaving out when we mix up formula or feed the baby already mixed formulas.

CHAPTER 32

Do Arthritics
Have a Deficiency
in Zinc?

THE WORD COLLAGEN is defined in the medical dictionary as "the albuminoid (protein) substance of the white fibers of connective tissues, cartilage and bone. It is converted into gelatin by boiling." So it includes all those body tissues which "hold us together." Irwin Stone, in his book *The Healing Factor, Vitamin C Against Disease*, defines collagen as "The main structural protein of the body, comprising about one-third of the protein content of the body. This is the cementing substance that holds the tissues and organs intact, forms and maintains the integrity of the vein and artery walls, lends strength and flexibility to the bones, and is the main component of scar tissue and healing wounds. The body cannot produce collagen without ascorbic acid (vitamin C). The most distressing symptoms of scurvy are caused by defective or absent collagen." Scurvy is the disease of vitamin C deficiency.

There is a close relationship between vitamin C and collagen. This relationship is what makes vitamin C so valuable in the performance of so many functions in the body. After all, if vitamin C, in given amounts, is necessary for producing and maintaining the health of everything in our bodies that connects everything to everything else, it surely must be involved with just about everything that goes well or goes wrong in our bodies.

All the various conditions that are grouped under the head of arthritic diseases are also called "collagen" diseases, since it is the connective tissue which is disordered or inadequate in these conditions.

Recently we came upon some information on the trace mineral zinc which seems to indicate that it, too, is extremely important in regard to collagen—its formation and its good health. A new book, volume I of a series called *Trace Elements in Human Health and Disease,* deals with the trace minerals zinc and copper.

In a chapter on collagen, the authors, Felix Fernandez-Madrid, Ananda S. Prasad and Donald Oberleas, discuss the effects of zinc deficiency on the creation of this connective tissue called collagen. They describe experiments which show that the effect of zinc deficiency on the manufacture of collagen is a generalized effect on the manufacture of protein and on the workings of nucleic acid, rather than a direct effect on the manufacture of collagen.

For example, deficiency in the trace mineral zinc produced (in laboratory rats) a great decrease in the amount of three amino acids or forms of protein in the skin of the animal. These three (glycine, proline and lysine) are especially important ingredients of collagen. So lack of zinc, resulting in a lack of these three kinds of protein, could be very important, indeed, to the health of the skin, as well as other tissues.

This suggests, does it not, that anybody with any kind of skin condition might notice improvement by simply increasing the zinc in his or her diet. It also suggests that the almost universal complaint of skin ailments these days—especially among teenagers—may have a lot to do with lack of zinc in their diets.

It is well known that wounds do not heal as quickly as they should in living things which are deficient in zinc. Giving zinc improves this situation. Zinc accumulates at the site of an injury, which seems to demonstrate that the body sends it there to help in healing, as white blood corpuscles are sent immediately to a wounded area to help in healing.

It is well known, too, that children who are deficient in zinc do not grow as they should, which seems to indicate that they do not have enough of this trace mineral to help them make the protein necessary for all the collagen in bones, cartilage and other connective tissues. "In general," say these authors, "studies of a variety of connective tissues in the zinc-deficient state have shown conclusively a significant reduction in the total collagen in the zinc deficient state."

People deficient in zinc also show abnormalities in the way the body uses those important substances DNA and RNA, which are the elements in cells which regulate heredity. As each cell divides, it takes with it part of the original RNA and DNA, so that the next cell will be normal. These substances are also made of protein. If zinc is essential in making protein, then it seems likely that the creation and operation of RNA and DNA (also called nucleic acids) would suffer.

It seems, indeed, from several reports, that zinc participates in the manufacture of nucleic acids—RNA and DNA. In animals made deficient in zinc the body manufacture of DNA was impaired. DNA is necessary for cells to divide. Cells must divide in order to create collagen. So the breakdown of this entire process seems to be implicated in reduction of collagen which develops in animals deficient in zinc.

There is every reason to believe that the same thing happens in human beings. Lack of zinc causes disordered collagen health and inefficient repair. Now think, for a moment, of the many parts of the body which are likely to suffer from such a circumstance. Most of all, think of the millions of Americans imprisoned in a "collagen disease" of one kind or another—rheumatoid arthritis, osteoarthritis, gout, lupus erythematosus, rheumatic heart disease in children, and so on, through the whole dismal catalog of ills.

Right now some three and a half million Americans suffer from some form of collagen disease. According to the Arthritis Foundation, about 97 per cent of all Americans over the age of 60 have collagen diseases of greater or less severity. In other words, these diseases are almost universal among older folks.

Doesn't it seem quite possible that one reason, at least, for this epidemic is the fact that practically all the zinc is removed from that group of foods which make up about half of most American diets—the refined carbohydrates—and is never replaced! Since these are the foods in which zinc is quite plentiful, it seems likely, does it not, that people who have eaten real wholegrain breads and cereals and have eliminated white sugar from their diets early in life are much less likely to suffer from the arthritic diseases than those who continue, throughout life, to eat white bread, exclusively, plus desserts, processed, sugary cereals, soft drinks, candy and so on, to the exclusion of most foods which contain any zinc at all.

In 1973, testifying before a Senate Select Committee, Dr. Walter Mertz, Chairman of Human Nutrition Institute of the U.S. Department of Agriculture, said, "We have not yet learned to understand the optimum requirement for all essential trace nutrients. Therefore, if we fabricate our own foods, we must accept that our knowledge is incomplete and therefore it is entirely possible that our fabricated foods are inferior in quality to that of the more wholesome products... we certainly have an example in zinc nutrition. In the past 5 to 10 years evidence has accumulated that the zinc nutrition status of a proportion of our older population is not optimal as shown by very good effects of increasing their zinc intake."

He went on to describe one of the commonest symptoms of zinc deficiency—lack of or impairment of a sense of taste. One survey showed that 8 to 10 per cent of supposedly normal children from middle and high income families were markedly deficient in zinc, as shown by the fact that their taste sensation was deficient, and they lacked appetite. Lack of appetite is very common among older folks. And often it is accompanied by the complaint, "I just don't seem to be able to taste anything any more." We quote more of Dr. Mertz's testimony on page 119.

No one, so far as we know, has correlated these complaints with arthritic disease. That is, we cannot prove that arthritics are deficient in zinc, since this lack of appetite and sense of taste is one of the chief symptoms of zinc deficiency. But why wait until someone performs all the laboratory work necessary to make such a deduction? Why not be sure to get enough zinc now, every day, in order to prevent arthritic diseases, if they threaten you, or perhaps alleviate them if you already have one or another of these painful conditions?

CHAPTER 33

There's Toxic Cadmium in Cigarette Smoke

THE HIGHLY TOXIC trace mineral cadmium has been suggested as a possible cause of high blood pressure. A recent investigation reported in *The Lancet* (December 4, 1976) found that there was no higher blood level of cadmium in 70 hypertensive patients than in those 70 people whose blood pressure was normal. However, the University of Glasgow researchers found that the level of cadmium in the blood of smokers was significantly higher than in the blood of non-smokers.

"The differences in blood-cadmium between smokers and non-smokers found here and elsewhere...confirm that cigarette smoke is an important source of cadmium to the body. Cigarette smokers do not have higher blood pressures than non-smokers, although they have increased cardiovascular mortality."

In the same issue of this medical journal an editorial points out that "it would be a dangerous oversimplification to consign cadmium to the dustbin of history: the present evidence suggests a complex situation in which certain forms of cadmium retention may have relevance to the raising of blood pressure."

The editorial goes on to describe cases of cadmium poisoning in Japan in which symptoms were bone disease, protein in the urine, and kidney failure. Cadmium is tightly bound by the kidney, says the *Lancet*, to such an extent that it is excreted only after long exposure. The observation that circulatory diseases are more prevalent where drinking water is "soft" may have nothing to do with the absence of the helpful minerals calcium and magnesium in the soft waters. Instead, the soft waters may leach cadmium into the drinking water and this toxic metal may be causing the circulatory problems. Some drugs given to combat high blood pressure can chelate trace minerals—that is, combine with them and hasten their excretion. These drugs may thus help the hypertensive by causing the excretion of the toxic metal cadmium from his body.

Although not nearly all the answers are in, we must remember to beware of cadmium, no matter what its source. Until quite recently in historical time there was no way for human beings to be exposed to it. Now it is being mined and used in many ways by industry. Our bodies, unable to evolve methods of excreting it in such a short time, are bound to suffer grievous harm if we continue to be exposed to it.

As we learned on page 223, one researcher has found high amounts of cadmium in lung tissue of smokers with emphysema. The severity of the disease is correlated with the length of time the patient has smoked. One cigarette contains about 1 microgram of cadmium. One pack deposits from 2 to 4 micrograms of cadmium in the smoker's lungs. Seventy per cent of the cadmium in tobacco passes into the smoke, which is inhaled or goes out into the room to be inhaled by everyone present, smokers and non-smokers alike. One researcher has calculated that the smoke from one pack of cigarettes, smoked over an eight-hour period in a 10′ by 12′ room releases over 100 times the amount of cadmium in the outside air.

Other sources of cadmium are air pollution from incinerators burning cadmium-containing products, such as rubber tires and plastic containers. Air and water pollution near refining plants of other metals, especially zinc, contains cadmium. The toxic metal has been found in almost half the drinking waters from rivers and reservoirs in the country. It accumulates in water stored in galvanized or plastic water pipes. Phosphate detergents may carry cadmium along with arsenic into our waterways.

Foods grown in soil heavily fertilized with phosphates pick up some cadmium which is a contaminant of the phosphates. Cadmium, much more toxic than lead, is present in old lead-based paint. The lead in the blood of children who eat paint flakes is also loaded with cadmium.

Cadmium is present in all gasolines. It goes into the engine's oils and becomes an air pollutant when these are burned. Various industries release cadmium into waterways. Fish caught near a battery factory on the Hudson River were recently found to be heavily contaminated with cadmium. Cadmium in grains is mostly in the starchy part—that part which remains in white flour and processed cereals when the germ and bran are removed. At the same time, zinc, which helps to protect us somewhat from the toxic effects of cadmium, is removed in the germ and bran. So people who eat only white bread and processed cereals have two strikes against them—too much cadmium and too little protective zinc, from their bread and cereals.

We recommend, of course, never smoking. If you are addicted to cigarettes, get over it, even if it means locking yourself in a room and going "cold turkey." Don't sit in a room where anyone is smoking, if you can possibly avoid it. Take zinc supplements in any case, since they may help to protect you against any cadmium to which you have been exposed.

CHAPTER 34

A Medical
Detective Story

A MYSTERY STORY involving arsenic in a sealant sold in a hardware store was related in *The New York Times* on December 29, 1976. Dr. James Darnell, a research scientist at the Rockefeller University, bought the silicon sealant to apply to the vinyl lining of his wife's dishwasher which had worn thin. Several months later Mrs. Darnell and her children began to suffer from symptoms which they thought were flu—nausea, stomach pains, low-grade fever and increasing weakness.

Tiny white translucent specks began to appear on the Darnell's dishes. A General Electric repairman made some repairs. The dishes continued to be spotted. By now muscle aching and hacking coughs had appeared in the Darnell family—except for Dr. Darnell who seldom ate at home. A second repairman, called in several months later, found that the sealant had not adhered to the lining of the dishwasher, but was flaking off and clinging to the dishes.

Mrs. Darnell set out to discover what was in the sealant. Nobody seemed to be able to tell her, until finally one GE official told her the product contained a very small amount of arsenic—"no more than you might eat in three shrimp." Dr. Darnell had the sealant analysed. It contained 25 times more arsenic than the GE official had mentioned.

The Darnell's doctor finally began to make tests. After

checking with an expert in the field, he told the Darnells they were suffering from arsenic poisoning. Mrs. Darnell and one of her sons had such high levels of arsenic in their tissues that they had to undergo a very painful treatment with the drug dimercaprol, which removes toxic arsenic, mercury and/or gold from the body. Medical bills for the entire incident were $10,000. The Darnells sued General Electric for $12 million and, at the time this story was written, they were preparing to settle out of court for $25,000, for they are weary of the five years of litigation they have been through.

No one is quite sure whether other symptons will develop in the future, especially in Mrs. Darnell and the one son who was most affected. Experts say that reaction to arsenic poisoning can be very variable—from "nothing to death." The sealant, which was also recommended on the label for mending china, contained no mention of possible danger except the brief warning that it should not be used in aquariums. The Darnells disposed of their china and silverware since the arsenic could not be removed.

Arsenic is used in herbicides, pesticides, wood preservatives, rat poisons. It is believed that one reason for lung cancer in smokers may be the arsenic which remains on the tobacco leaves after they are sprayed with pesticides. Arsenic is a contaminant of phosphate detergents and is washed into waterways in the sewage which carries away the detergents. Several years ago the Department of Agriculture warned us that arsenic was appearing in very small amounts in the livers of some animals which we eat. The USDA experts assured us that this was a form of arsenic which is not "very toxic."

Nevertheless, it's something to keep in mind. And it's well to check as carefully as you can on any household chemicals you use which may come into contact with food. If it's at all possible avoid using a new product about which you feel uncertain—don't use it. Medical detective stories don't always end happily.

CHAPTER 35

Zinc Supplements
Clear Up
Acne Problems

CERTAIN CHEMICAL FORMS of vitamin A have been prescribed successfully by some American physicians in the treatment of acne. Now we read of several Swedish physicians who are using vitamin A and the mineral zinc to treat this unsightly skin disease. According to *Archives of Dermatology* for January 1977, Dr. G. Michaelsson and his colleagues gave zinc sulfate in very large doses (135 milligrams daily) alone and in combination with vitamin A. The results were compared with results from vitamin A alone and a pill containing nothing.

To decide just how effective each of these treatments was, the doctors counted the number of "pimples" at each visit. After four weeks there was a significant decrease in the number of such skin flaws in the group taking zinc. Those taking zinc and vitamin A got no better score. And the group taking the "nothing" pill showed no change.

Most important of all, after 12 weeks of treatment the score on numbers of pimples had decreased from 100 per cent to 15 per cent. It seems to us that any teenager should welcome such a treatment with glee, and should persist in it until he or she completely clears those ugly pustules from the skin.

We have emphasized many times our conviction, bulwarked by a great deal of significant research, that acne is caused by the consumption of too much refined carbohydrate—that is, too much white sugar and white flour and foods made from them. No one seems to know just why this diet should cause acne, although teenagers in primitive countries who do not have access to these foods never suffer from this disease.

Now it seems that lack of zinc, caused by the diet high in refined carbohydrate, may be the chief cause of acne. As we know, all the zinc has been removed from sugar cane when it is refined into white sugar. And all the zinc is removed from white flour and processed cereals when they are refined into the satiny, white fluffy stuff called white flour and the crispy, crunchy, sugary stuff in the supermarket cereal boxes.

Zinc is essential for processing carbohydrate foods. It is vitally involved in regulating blood sugar levels which are usually deranged by diets high in sugar and refined starch. so perhaps it is indeed the lack of zinc, along with lack of the B vitamins (also necessary for the body to process sugar and starch) which brings on acne.

In any case, it's an easy treatment to try for oneself. The Swedish doctors gave 135 milligrams of zinc as zinc sulfate. That is, the pills contained more than 135 milligrams, but they provided that much zinc every day. No mention is made of any change in diet, but it goes without saying that improvement would certainly be noticed much sooner by someone taking the zinc, and also revising meals and snacks so that sugary and starchy goodies are eliminated.

Why not try it, if you are bothered by acne? The diet to follow is very simple: eat only meat, fish, poultry, dairy products, all vegetables and fruits in any quantity, plus real wholegrain breads and cereals, seeds and nuts. And nothing more. No sugar in any form. No soft drinks, no candy, no desserts except fruit. Zinc is available at your health food store in many preparations. Space the tablets out through the day taking them with each meal rather than taking them all at once. A chelated zinc preparation will probably make absorption of the mineral more certain. And of course continue to take your usual vitamin and mineral supplements every day as, we hope, you always do.

CHAPTER 36

Zinc Therapy for Sickle-Cell Anemia

SICKLE-CELL ANEMIA is a devastating disease in which a large number of red blood cells are deformed to resemble sickles or crescents. The resulting anemia may cause blood clots, heart attacks, liver problems, painful arthritis with fever, ulcers around the ankles, episodes of severe stomach pain and vomiting, plus many kinds of nerve disorders. Amost every part of the body suffers when something is the matter with blood cells.

Victims of sickle-cell anemia are usually poorly developed—that is, they do not grow properly and their bones are not normal. Because of this peculiarity, a specialist in trace minerals may have discovered a treatment for this form of anemia which can possibly arrest it or, who knows, prevent it.

Dr. Ananda S. Prasad, professor of medicine at Wayne State University in Detroit, has turned up a great deal of evidence on growth abnormalities caused by zinc deficiency. Giving zinc to some people suffering from dwarfism has encouraged additional growth. Dr. Prasad decided to try zinc on sickle-cell patients to see if he might be able to help their growth problems. He did. And in the process he discovered that their leg ulcers healed, their sex organs became more normal.

Dr. George J. Brewer of the University of Michigan carried these studies further by also giving zinc supplements to sickle cell patients. He discovered that he could actually improve the condition of the blood cells. He gave his patients massive doses of zinc acetate. Every four hours, day and night, they took zinc until they were taking a total of 150 milligrams. He got a 10 per cent improvement in hemoglobin (red blood cells), numbers of red blood cells and survival of red blood cells.

"If this had been the sole beneficial effect," he says in an article in a January 1977 issue of *Medical World News*, "it would be too small to justify therapy of this complexity." But these were not the only effects of the zinc therapy. Ten patients who took zinc had been suffering from an average of about 6 pain episodes a year. Zinc therapy cut this down to about 2.3 episodes.

Furthermore, the zinc cut down the number of irreversibly sickled cells, those red blood cells so badly damaged that they cannot be brought back to a healthy state. But the number of these cells decreased after zinc therapy. The count actually went down from 28 per cent to 18.6 per cent. It is believed that the actual number of sickled blood cells governs the amount of damage that may be done to blood vessels and spleen. So presumably any decrease in the number of such cells would improve the general condition of the patient.

A group of scientists at the University of Minnesota headed by Dr. John W. Eaton is looking into another aspect of minerals in relation to sickle-cell anemia. He has found, he says, that sickled cells contain abnormal amounts of calcium. This is especially true of the cells that are irreversibly damaged. So something appears to be wrong with the way the bodies of these patients are using calcium. This, too, may be related to zinc. Dr. Eaton found that zinc can partially block the entrance of excessive amounts of calcium into the diseased cells.

Dr. Brewer thinks that zinc benefits the membrane of the sickled cell by somehow opposing the damage done by excessive calcium but he does not know as yet just how the whole thing works. At any rate, it looks very promising for future research which may be able to devise a way to use zinc so that further degeneration of the patient's blood may be arrested. Or, it seems to us, such a trend in research may produce some astonishing insights into what causes this disease. It is hereditary. It is found almost exclusively in Blacks. Might the original injury which caused the hereditary condition not be related to a lifetime deficiency in zinc?

We do not know. Undoubtedly any such discoveries are far in the future. Part of the reason why any therapy with zinc is difficult is the way the supplement must be given. Investigators have found that the amount of zinc in an individual's blood rises to a peak about two hours after he takes a zinc supplement. Then it goes down to its former level in about five hours. So the zinc must be taken in very small doses every four hours around the clock, which is a difficult and inconvenient schedule to maintain.

Few patients with a serious case of sickle-cell anemia live beyond the age of 40. Infections (TB for example), blood clots in the lungs or in some other vital area are usually the cause of death. Any harmless therapy, such as zinc therapy, which can do anything to alleviate the sickling of blood cells which produces the disease is certainly a ray of hope, since no other therapy is known.

Researchers trying to solve one physiological mystery must, it seems, confine themselves to a study of only one element—zinc in this case. What great advances might be made in understanding this disorder if scientists would use, in addition to the zinc, the best possible diet, as highly nutritious as could be devised, along with supplements of all the vitamins and all the minerals known to be essential!

Suggested Further Reading

Adams, Ruth and Frank Murray, *The High Risks of a Low Calcium Diet*, Larchmont Books, New York, 1972.

Ellis, John M., *Vitamin B6, the Doctor's Report*, Harper and Row, New York, 1973.

Food, The Yearbook of Agriculture 1959, The U.S. Department of Agriculture, Washington, D.C.

The Heinz Handbook of Nutrition, McGraw-Hill Book Co., Inc., London, New York, Toronto, 1959.

Hemphill, Delbert D., Editor, *Trace Substances in Environmental Health*, Volume V., University of Missouri, Columbia, 1972.

Holvey, David M., Editor, *The Merck Manual of Diagnosis and Therapy*, Merck and Co., Inc., Rahway, N.J., 1972.

Lee, Douglas H.K., Editor, *Metallic Contaminants and Human Health*, Academic Press, New York and London, 1972.

Modell, Walter, *Drugs in Current Use*, Springer Publishing Co., New York, 1962.

Monier-Williams, G.W., *Trace Elements in Food*, John Wiley and Sons, Inc., New York, 1949.

Price, Dr. Joseph M., *Coronaries, Cholesterol & Chlorine*, Pyramid Books, New York, 1972.

Schroeder, Henry A., *Pollution, Profits and Progress*, The Stephen Greene Press, Brattleboro, Vermont, 1971.

Schroeder, Henry A., *The Trace Elements and Man*, Devin-Adair Company, Old Greenwich, Conn., 1974.

Schütte, Karl H., *The Biology of the Trace Elements*, J. B. Lippincott Company, Philadelphia and Montreal, 1964.

Underwood, E. J., *Trace Elements in Human and Animal Nutrition*, 3rd Edition, Academic Press, New York and London, 1971.

Waldbott, G. L., *Health Effects of Environmental Pollutants*, C. V. Mosby, St. Louis, 1973.

Index

Ferrous sulfate, 100
Fertilizers, commercial, 25, 33, 52, 151, 157, 226, 231, 233, 264 ff.
Fieve, Dr. Ronald R., 185, 191
Fingernails, 70, 154, 232
Fingers, pain in, 114
Fischer, Dr. Richard P., 234
Fish, lead and mercury poisoning of, 235 ff., 250
Fish and shellfish, nutrients in, 90
Fitness for Living, 156
Flour, white, 25
Fluoridation, 45, 47, 196 ff., 281
Fluoride, 13, 27, 47, 196 ff., 248, 268, 280,
Fluoride poisoning, 199, 200, 203, 205, 206, 208, 209
Fluorine, 20, 45, 49, 209, 268
Folic acid, a B vitamin, 97, 116, 125, 127, 331
Food, U.S. Department of Agriculture Yearbook, 12, 57, 71, 76, 80, 86, 110, 132, 141, 144
Food and Drug Administration, 11, 18, 27, 68, 100, 103, 142, 178, 207, 218, 236, 245, 302,
Food for Us All, 86
Food in History, 296
Foods, absorption of nutrients in, 96, 98, 103, 121, 150, 220
Foods, frozen, 143
Foods, imbalances in, 116
Foods, unrefined and unprocessed, 16, 46
Food Technology, 299
Forman, Dr. Jonathan, 209
Fouad, Dr. M. Taher, 280
Friedlander, Dr. S. K., 246
Fruit juice, 145

G

Gallium, 54
Garrison, Dr. Glen E., 140
Gasoline, cadmium and lead in, 226, 245
Gelatin, 70, 232
Genetics, 30, 43, 102
George Washington Law Review, 212
Geriatrics, 138

Germanium, 259
Gillespie, Dr. S. M., 205
Glasgow, University of, 339
Glucose tolerance factor, 161, 164, 314,
Glucose tolerance test, 19
Goat's milk, 72
Goiter, 12, 21, 23, 27, 41, 55, 86, 192, 205, 233, 247, 306
Goldberg, Dr. Alan M., 254
Gordus, Dr. Adon A., 156
Gormican, Dr. Annette, 32
Gout, 187
Goya, Francisco de, 244
GP, 208
Graff, Dr. Darrel, 284
Grains, whole, 93, 94, 106
Griggs, Kyle, 217
Guinee, Dr. Vincent, 251
Gums, 71, 94
Gunther, Dr. Mavis, 330

H

Hair, color of, 23, 125, 151
Hair, loss of, 112
Hair, mineral analysis of, 290
Hair, mineral content of, 31, 39, 124, 156, 163, 233, 255, 282,
Hambridge, K. M., 156
Hammer, Dr. D. I., 40
Hardening of the arteries, 14, 112, 123, 125, 162, 166
Hardy, Dr. Harriet L., 227
Harvard University, 119, 220, 262
Hathaway, Milicent L., 57
The Healing Factor, Vitamin C Against Disease, 334
Health care, costs for, 32
Health Effects of Environmental Pollutants, 218
Health food stores, 55, 70, 72, 74, 85, 105, 106, 139, 143, 277, 280,
Heart, 58, 71, 110, 122, 133
Heart disease, 13, 14, 15, 31, 35, 36, 37, 38, 109, 112, 114, 116, 139, 145, 146, 148, 170, 180, 198, 227
Heinz Handbook of Nutrition, 87
Helmer, Prof. O. M., 135
Hemochromatosis, 102

FOOD AND NUTRITION BOARD, NATIONAL ACADEMY OF SCIENCES—NATIONAL RESEARCH COUNCIL RECOMMENDED DAILY DIETARY ALLOWANCES. Revised 1974

AGE (years)	WEIGHT (kg)	WEIGHT (lbs)	HEIGHT (cm)	HEIGHT (in)	ENERGY (kcal)	PROTEIN (g)	VITAMIN A ACTIVITY (IU)	(IU)	VITAMIN D (IU)	VITAMIN E ACTIVITY (IU)
Infants										
0.0-0.5	6	14	60	24	kg x 117	kg x 2.2	420	1,400	400	4
0.5-1.0	9	20	71	28	kg x 108	kg x 2.0	400	2,000	400	5
Children										
1-3	13	28	86	34	1,300	23	400	2,000	400	7
4-6	20	44	110	44	1,800	30	500	2,500	400	9
7-10	30	66	135	54	2,400	36	700	3,300	400	10
Males										
11-14	44	97	158	63	2,800	44	1,000	5,000	400	12
15-18	61	134	172	69	3,000	54	1,000	5,000	400	15
19-22	67	147	172	69	3,000	54	1,000	5,000	400	15
23-50	70	154	172	69	2,700	56	1,000	5,000		15
51+	70	154	172	69	2,400	56	1,000	5,000		15
Females										
11-14	44	97	155	62	2,400	44	800	4,000	400	12
15-18	54	119	162	65	2,100	46	800	4,000	400	12
19-22	58	128	162	65	2,100	46	800	4,000	400	12
23-50	58	128	162	65	2,000	46	800	4,000		12
51+	58	128	162	65	1,800	46	800	4,000		12
Pregnant					+300	+30	1,000	5,000	400	15
Lactating					+500	+20	1,200	6,000	400	15

a The allowances are intended to provide for individual variations among most normal persons as they live in the United States under usual environmental stresses. Diets should be based on a variety of common foods in order to provide other nutrients for which human requirements have been less well defined. See text for more detailed discussion of allowances and of nutrients not tabulated. See Table I (p. 6) for weights and heights by individual year of age.

b Kilojoules (kJ) = 4.2 × kcal.

c Retinol equivalents.

d Assumed to be all as retinol in milk during the first six months of life. All subsequent intakes are assumed to be half as retinol and half as B-carotene when calculated from

364

Designed for the maintenance of good nutrition of practically all healthy people in the U.S.A.

| | WATER-SOLUBLE VITAMINS | | | | | | | MINERALS | | | | |
Ascorbic Acid (mg)	Folacin (µg)	Niacin (mg)	Riboflavin (mg)	Thiamin (mg)	Vitamin B6 (mg)	Vitamin B12 (µg)	Calcium (mg)	Phosphorus (mg)	Iodine (µg)	Iron (mg)	Magnesium (mg)	Zinc (mg)
35	50	5	0.4	0.3	0.3	0.3	360	240	35	10	60	3
35	50	8	0.6	0.5	0.4	0.3	540	400	45	15	70	5
40	100	9	0.8	0.7	0.6	1.0	800	800	60	15	150	10
40	200	12	1.1	0.9	0.9	1.5	800	800	80	10	200	10
40	300	16	1.2	1.2	1.2	2.0	800	800	110	10	250	10
45	400	18	1.5	1.4	1.6	3.0	1,200	1,200	130	18	350	15
45	400	20	1.8	1.5	2.0	3.0	1,200	1,200	150	18	400	15
45	400	20	1.8	1.5	2.0	3.0	800	800	140	10	350	15
45	400	18	1.6	1.4	2.0	3.0	800	800	130	10	350	15
45	400	16	1.5	1.2	2.0	3.0	800	800	110	10	350	15
45	400	16	1.3	1.2	1.6	3.0	1,200	1,200	115	18	300	15
45	400	14	1.4	1.1	2.0	3.0	1,200	1,200	115	18	300	15
45	400	14	1.4	1.1	2.0	3.0	800	800	100	18	300	15
45	400	13	1.2	1.0	2.0	3.0	800	800	100	18	300	15
45	400	12	1.1	1.0	2.0	3.0	800	800	80	10	300	15
60	800	+2	+0.3	+0.3	2.5	4.0	1,200	1,200	125	18+	450	20
80	600	+4	+0.5	+0.3	2.5	4.0	1,200	1,200	150	18	450	25

international units. As retinol equivalents, three fourths are as retinol and one fourth as B-carotene.

c Total vitamin E activity, estimated to be 80 percent as a-tocopherol and 20 percent other tocopherols. See text for variation in allowances.

f The folacin allowances refer to dietary sources as determined by *Lactobacillus casei* assay. Pure forms of folacin may be effective in doses less than one fourth of the recommended dietary allowance.

g Although allowances are expressed as niacin, it is recognized that on the average 1 mg of niacin is derived from each 60 mg of dietary tryptophan.

h This increased requirement cannot be met by ordinary diets; therefore, the use of supplemental iron is recommended.

*The best books on health and
nutrition are from*

LARCHMONT BOOKS

10) Too much fluoride can cause tooth mottling and allergies?

11) There is now a Recommended Dietary Allowance for zinc?

12) Hyperactive children often have raised levels of lead in their blood?

13) Plutonium, used at some nuclear power plants, is the single most toxic material in the world?

14) Chelated minerals can harmlessly purge your system of toxic compounds?

15) Over one-fourth of American children have levels of lead in their bodies that border on toxicity?

16) 43 trace elements may be ingredients in tooth enamel?

17) Too much bed rest depletes your calcium stores?

18) An iodine deficiency causes goiter?

19) Women often lose considerable amounts of iron in menstrual flow?

20) Vitamin E and selenium are related?

21) A molybdenum deficiency can cause cancer of the digestive tract?

22) Chronic beryllium poisoning may not develop until 25 years after exposure?

23) Cadmium—a greater threat to health than lead and mercury—can cause high blood pressure and kidney and liver damage?

24) A chromium and vitamin B6 deficiency may cause hardening of the arteries?

25) Vitamin B12 contains two metals—cobalt and phosphorus?

26) Copper and zinc may affect the color of your hair?

27) Chlorine—which destroys vitamin E—may cause heart attacks?

28) Calcium, magnesium, potassium and vitamin B6 may prevent leg cramps?

29) About one-third of American women over 50 have osteoporosis, a calcium deficiency disorder?

30) Calcium, zinc and vanadium may lower cholesterol levels?